THE
COLLEGE DORM
WORKOUT ▬▬▬

THE
COLLEGE DORM
WORKOUT

*Fight the Freshman Fifteen
in Twenty Minutes a Day
without Starving to Death*

MARTHE SIMONE VEDRAL
AND JOYCE L. VEDRAL, PH.D.

WARNER BOOKS

A Time Warner Company

This book is not intended as a substitute for medical advice. The reader should regularly consult a physician in matters relating to his or her health and particularly with respect to any symptoms that may require diagnosis or medical attention.

Copyright © 1994 by Marthe S. Vedral and Joyce L. Vedral, Ph.D.
All rights reserved.

Warner Books, Inc., 1271 Avenue of the Americas, New York, NY 10020

A Time Warner Company

Printed in the United States of America

First Printing: January 1994

10 9 8 7 6 5 4 3 2 1

Library of Congress Cataloging-in-Publication Data

Vedral, Marthe.
The college dorm workout / Marthe Vedral and Joyce Vedral.
p.   cm.
Includes index.
ISBN 0-446-39477-7
1. Exercise.   2. Physical fitness.   I. Vedral, Joyce L.
II. Title.
GV481.W43   1994
613.7'1—dc20   93-17617   CIP

Cover outfit by Capezio from Ballet Makers, Inc.

Cover photo and interior photos by Don Banks

Bathing suits by Nicole Gangi, of Nicole's Perfect Fit, Glen Cove, New York

Leotards for opening chapters by Capezio from Ballet Makers, Inc.

Workout leotard by Dance France

Gym shoes by Reebok International

Hair and makeup by Jody Pollutro

Book design by Giorgetta Bell McRee

Cover design by Diane Luger

To every college student who wishes to be free,
once and for all, of the worries
about weight gain and shape!

CONTENTS

ACKNOWLEDGMENTS

To Joann Davis, for making this project happen.

To Pam Bernstein, our agent, for working out "the deal."

To Jeanmarie, for your careful work on the manuscript.

To Diane Luger and Jackie Merri Meyer, for your creativity in the cover art.

To Larry Kirshbaum, Nanscy Neiman, and Ellen Herrick, for your continual enthusiasm and support.

To Edna Farley, for your talented handling of the publicity.

To Don Banks, for your wonderful photography.

To Jody Pollutro, for fantastic hair and makeup.

To family and friends, for your continual love and support.

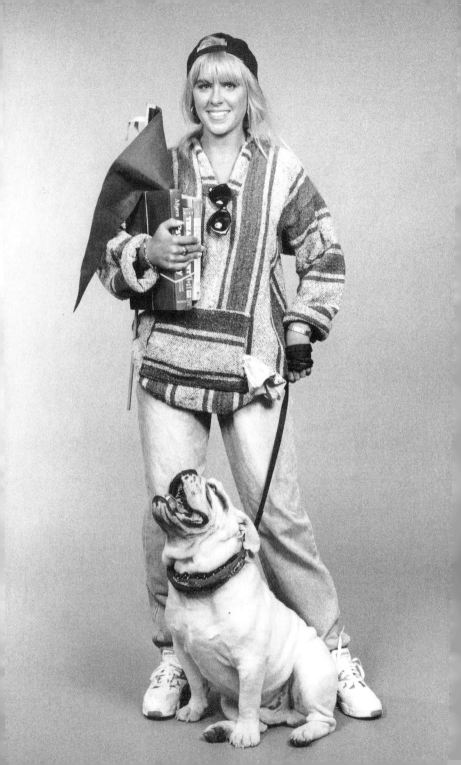

YOU DON'T HAVE TO GET (OR STAY) FAT JUST BECAUSE YOU'RE IN COLLEGE!

You've worked and you've planned, and finally you made it. You're in college. You're worried about getting good grades. You're hoping to meet some interesting people. You may be wondering if you'll be able to make the adjustment—being away from home. In other words, you've got plenty to deal with. The last thing in the world you need to worry about is getting fat!

But it happens. It happens gradually—and at first you don't realize it—not until your clothes start to feel a little tight, and you find yourself wearing baggy sweats more and more—and you notice that, mysteriously, so are many other girls that used to wear clothes to show off their figures.

You're not alone—the problem is common, in fact, so common that the phrase "freshman fifteen" has been coined. But that's small comfort to you. You don't want to

1

be fat just because you're in college—and you don't have to be. Not only can you be your ideal size, but you can have shape, definition, and just the right-sized muscles so that you will look better than you ever did in your life.

WHY DO PEOPLE GAIN WEIGHT IN COLLEGE?

It's the easiest thing in the world to gain fifteen pounds in your first year of college, and to keep those pounds throughout your college career—even adding more as you go along. The reason for this is quite simple: change of diet and activity level, and falling into some of the not-so-obvious traps of college living and college social life.

College menus are replete with fat-laden foods, and unless you know exactly how to pick, choose, and avoid and even supplement certain foods, you can gain a steady pound or two a week. And to make things even worse, if you're feeling a little homesick, you may get into the habit of consoling yourself with double and triple portions of dessert.

When it comes to activity, although there is plenty to do on campus besides study, a certain amount of studying must be done—and since this involves sitting in a chair or lying on a bed rather than moving around, it's easy enough to begin to see a hip spread. Also, if you're living on campus, chances are you don't walk as much as before, because everything is conveniently located. Or you may get into your car and drive everywhere.

And last, but certainly not least, there's college life in general—social life and campus living. Much of the drinking and eating in college are a part of meeting and getting to know new people. The keg parties, the 3:00 A.M. pizza binges, and the all-nighters when you're cramming for an exam and use junk food to keep you going—these occasions all pose dangers to your shape.

Whether you have gained weight because of one or all of the above, or whether you haven't gained weight yet but are afraid you will, or even if you are not overweight but just want to get into better shape, this book is for you. It will show you how to participate fully in college life—without falling into the above traps; and what's more, it will give you a workout that will give you the body of your dreams—and in only twenty minutes a day with exercises that you can do in the privacy of your own room, no matter how small that room may be.

IT HAPPENED TO ME!

When I (Marthe) first arrived at college, I never dreamed that I would have a weight problem, yet in my first semester I gained nearly fifteen pounds—for all of the reasons listed above. I found myself doing an awful lot of shopping for clothing—not because I had money to spare, but rather because nothing looked right in the mirror.

In a panic, I tried starving myself, and when that didn't work, I resorted to a liquid diet that caused me to be so desperate that one day I ripped open a box of chocolates that I had bought someone as a gift and ate the whole thing in a matter of minutes. In despair, I continued to try different things. I even started running around the track every day, but nothing worked—until ...

TEN WEEKS TO ZAP THE FRESHMAN FIFTEEN

I decided to ask my mom, who as you may already know is a well-known fitness expert. She's trained with champion bodybuilders and has written for *Muscle and Fitness* and *Shape* magazines for years. In addition, she is the author of the *New York Times* bestselling book *The Fat-Burning Workout*, and more recently, *Gut Busters* and *Bottoms Up!* Together, we worked out a system that could be used by college students who have only the limited space of their cramped dorm rooms—even rooms with as little as four feet of floor space in length and two feet in width. What's more, we figured out a way to condense the workout into twenty minutes. We also put together a realistic eating plan that allows you to eat plenty of low-fat foods (yes, even within the horrible limitations of most college menus). The foundation of our plan is taken from time-honored secrets of champion bodybuilders.

First, I applied this system to myself, and in six weeks I had lost ten pounds and toned up my body, and in another four, I lost the last five pounds. Now, for the first time in my life, I'm in the shape I always dreamed of—but more important, I've been able to get hundreds of other college girls in shape too!

WHAT YOU CAN EXPECT FROM THIS PROGRAM

Now let me tell you about the goals of the college dorm workout. If you follow this program, you can expect to:

- Lose ten to fifteen pounds in six to ten weeks
- Go down a size in jeans in three weeks
- Attain perfectly formed muscles in all the right places
- Acquire knowledge of how to work around the college menu so that you can eat plenty without getting fat
- Achieve peace of mind once and for all regarding your weight and the shape of your body
- Increase your metabolism so you can eat more without getting fat
- Improve your posture
- Increase your self-discipline and self-confidence
- Achieve a healthier heart and greater lung capacity
- Improve your performance in sports through greater strength and aerobic fitness
- Increase your ability to concentrate on your studies
- Relieve stress caused by studying, exams, and term papers.

ONLY TWENTY MINUTES A DAY

The best part of this program is it's streamlined. You don't have to spend hours working out. Since it's derived from the time-tested methods of champion bodybuilders and scientifically formulated to get the maximum results in the minimum of time, it's a condensed method of getting in shape. You work fast, and you work right.

Bodybuilders know the secrets of losing body fat and shaping perfect muscle. It's their life. If they don't have a perfect quadriceps (thigh) muscle or perfect "glutes" (buttocks muscles), for example, they can lose a contest. They know how to go back to the gym to create shapely muscles and get rid of fat on every part of the body. These secrets are contained in this book. They will reshape your body in record time.

THE SECRET OF THIS WORKOUT

The secret of this workout is its intensity. In just twenty minutes a day, you will really be getting a forty-minute workout because you are allowed very few rests, and because you apply continual pressure as you perform the movements. The end result is a workout that takes half the time and is more than twice as effective as other fitness routines. You not only burn more fat because of the speed of the workout, but you also get harder, more defined muscles because you are applying continual tension as you move.

To put it bluntly, with this workout, you will get more results in twenty minutes than most people only get after an hour of working out. The fact is, it's not the time you put in, but what you do in that time!

BUT WILL I LOOK LIKE A MUSCLE-BOUND BODYBUILDER?

Don't worry. You won't look like Arnold Schwarzenegger. In order to do that, you would have to work with heavy weights, and exercise for two to three hours a day. You will be using one simple set of five-pound dumbbells, and you will be developing perfectly shaped muscles in all the right places.

WHAT IS INVOLVED IN THIS PROGRAM?

You will be working out four to seven days a week. You will work out four days with weights, and then decide whether you want to use the extra three days to do an aerobic activity, to rest, or to do some additional work with weights. This will be discussed in Chapter 3. But whether you choose to work out four days a week or to speed up your progress by exercising seven days a week, you will get in shape and stay that way—because you will have discovered a program that will work for you for the rest of your life.

DO IT IN YOUR DORM WITH ONLY ONE SET OF DUMBBELLS!

Perhaps the best thing about this workout is you need almost no equipment to do it, and you don't have to go anywhere to do it. You do the workout in your dorm, with a set of three- or five-pound dumbbells. (You can buy them in any sporting goods store, or you can order them from us. See page 191). You don't need much space either. If you can sit in a chair, stand up, or lie on the floor, you have all the space you need.

Your workout will be fully explained in Chapter 3, but here is a quick overview of the basic workout—plans A and B.

Plan A		Plan B	
Sunday	Aerobic option or rest	Sunday	Rest
Monday	Upper body	Monday	Upper body
Tuesday	Lower body	Tuesday	Lower body
Wednesday	Aerobic option or rest	Wednesday	Upper body
Thursday	Upper body	Thursday	Lower body
Friday	Lower body	Friday	Upper body
Saturday	Aerobic option or rest	Saturday	Lower body

The reason you are allowed to choose between A and B is simple. *The College Dorm Workout* has a fat-burning, heart-and-lung-strengthening aerobic effect, so if you don't like aerobics, you can skip them and do additional weight workouts. On the other hand, if you love aerobics, and perhaps are already doing some aerobic activity, you can simply incorporate them into your workout.

HOW DOES THIS WORKOUT DIFFER FROM OTHER FITNESS PROGRAMS?

Regular bodybuilding. The College Dorm Workout utilizes the basic principles of bodybuilding (the split routine, muscle isolation, continual tension, and so forth—these terms will be explained in Chapter 2). The difference between this program and that of regular bodybuilding is that bodybuilders use much heavier weights and take longer rests. They also work for much longer periods of time—two to three hours a day. The end result is bodybuilders create huge, hulking muscles. Since you will be using much lighter weights, moving faster, and putting in less time, you will get much smaller muscles. In other words, if you follow this workout, there's no danger of you looking like the gigantic female bodybuilders you might have seen on television or in the magazines.

Nautilus and circuit training. In Nautilus and other circuit training, the exerciser works the entire body in one training session, as she advances from one machine ("station") to the next. The goal of this type of training is to develop muscle tone and to get an aerobic effect at the same time. Typically, only one set (a set is a group of repetitions) of one or two exercises are performed for each body part. The trouble with this workout, however, is you can never reshape your body by doing only one or two sets of exercise per body part. You must do a minimum of nine sets (as set forth in this workout) in order to challenge the muscle to the point where it will grow and be reshaped.

I'll never forget how frustrating it was for me while a high school senior, working part-time in a popular health spa. The manager told me to put the people on the "circuit," and when I explained to him that they would never get in shape that way, he said, "I know. I'm a bodybuilder myself. But we don't want them staying on one piece of equipment for too long. We have to keep them moving." I had to quit that job because it upset me to tell people to do something that would not work—when I knew what did work.

All that circuit training accomplishes is to burn some fat and to stimulate the muscle a little. The College Dorm Workout succeeds where circuit training fails. It provides an aerobic effect because you are working fast, but it also reshapes your muscle because you are challenging the muscle significantly.

Machines versus free weights. All well and good. But what about machines? Aren't they more effective than free weights such as the dumbbells you will use for this workout? The answer is definitely no. Machines are important if you are lifting very heavy weights, because if you should drop the weight, the machine would catch it for you and you wouldn't get hurt. In addition, machines are psychologically comforting. When you place yourself in the seat of a machine, you feel as if you are not alone, as if you are not doing all of the work—and indeed you are not. You see, machines allow you to cheat more, because as mentioned above, if you drop or half drop the weight, the machine will catch it.

Free weights, on the other hand, such as the dumbbells you will be using for this workout, force you to do all of the work. You are in complete control at all times, and you know it. Every inch of movement is performed by you and you alone. You get the most out of your workout time with free weights.

But what's even more important, you can do with one simple set of dumbbells what it would take many machines to do. For example, if you were to go to a gym and rely upon machines for the workout you are doing in this book, you would have to use bench press and pec-deck machines for your chest routine, shoulder press and shoulder lateral machines for your shoulder routine, biceps curl and triceps press machines for your arm routine, the lat pulldown and the pulley row machines for your back routine, the squat machine and the leg press machine for your thigh routine, the adductor and abductor machines for your buttocks routine, and the crunch and sit-up machines for your abdominals routine. You would need fourteen machines in all to do what *a simple pair of dumbbells could do better.*

If you don't believe that free weights are more effective than machines, observe any bodybuilder in a gym. You will note that most of his or her workout is comprised of free weights. (There are some useful machines, but that is a discussion for another time.)

WHY NOT USE AEROBICS ALONE?

An aerobic exercise is an activity that involves the major muscle groups and keeps your pulse rate between 60 percent and 85 percent of capacity for twenty minutes or longer. (You can figure out your maximum pulse rate by subtracting your age from 220. For example, if you are twenty years old, your maximum pulse rate is 200. If you keep your pulse 60 percent to 85 percent of 200 for twenty minutes, you get an aerobic, heart-and-lung-challenging, fat-burning effect.) The College Dorm Workout has an aerobic effect, because you keep your pulse rate up to about 60 percent to 70 percent of capacity throughout the workout.

Straight aerobic exercises that do not involve weight training are bike riding, running, swimming, rope jumping, walking fast, stair stepping, aerobic dance, and so on. While these activities are excellent for burning fat and helping to condition the heart and lungs, *they cannot reshape the entire body.* The most one could expect from an aerobic activity is some shaping of the body part involved in the workout. For example, swimmers will often have lovely V-shaped backs, and runners will have muscular legs—but both can have protruding stomachs and out-of-shape arms. Only working with weights the right way can reshape each body part into its perfect form.

WHY NOT SIMPLY DEPEND ON SPORTS AND GAMES TO STAY IN SHAPE

Since a sport is dependent upon the nature of the game, the actions of the opponent, and the skill of the player, and because they are not usually performed four or more times a week, sports cannot be depended upon either to consistently burn fat or to reshape the entire body. Of course, a sport will help to burn some calories and to reshape certain body parts. For example, a tennis player will have a well-developed forearm, and a soccer player will have great thighs. But neither the tennis player nor the soccer player may have gorgeous abdominal muscles.

And so it goes. The fact is, it's foolish to hope that your sport will be able to perfect your body shape. Only working with weights the right way can do that.

WHY DIETING ALONE WON'T DO IT!

You can lose weight—and indeed fat—by dieting, but you can't reshape your body by diet. As medical experts agree, it's very difficult to keep fat off your body by diet alone. You have to work out with weights to do that.

Working with weights the right way, for twenty minutes a day, will not only perfect the shape of every part of your body, but will build you feminine, perfectly formed muscle in all the right places, and these muscles will themselves help you to lose more weight.

MUSCLE BURNS FAT

Muscle is the only body material that is active. That is to say, when you have more muscle on your body, you raise your metabolism, so that whether you are sleeping, sitting in a chair, or standing up, you burn about 10 percent to 20 percent or more calories than you burned before— doing the same thing. The end result is you don't have to starve yourself to keep the fat off your body. In other words, once you have muscle, you can eat more than you did before without getting fat. In fact, *adding muscle to your body is the only sure way of losing weight and keeping it off* without resorting to extreme diets and/or obsessive and exhausting exercise programs.

HOW YOU CAN LOSE WEIGHT AND GET IN SHAPE WITHOUT STARVING YOURSELF TO DEATH

In order to lose excess body fat, or to put it another way, in order to lose weight, you must create a calorie deficit. For every 3,500 calories that are in deficit, your body gives up one pound of fat. There are two ways to create a calorie deficit: 1) By eating less food than your body burns during the course of a day. 2) By burning more energy and using up more calories than your body has been supplied.

Trying to lose weight by starvation dieting is self-defeating, because if your caloric intake goes below 1,000, your metabolism slows down and you burn fewer calories than you would have burned had you eaten more food and worked out. In addition, if you just diet and don't work out, you will eventually become a "skinny-fat." You may be bone thin, but your body will not be tight and toned.

There's no way around it. In order to lose weight, you have to do both—decrease your caloric intake not by starving, but by eating plenty of the right foods and avoiding high-fat foods, and also by working out with weights in order to put muscles on your body, muscles that in and of themselves burn fat twenty-four hours a day!

As you do the twenty-minute workout, you'll create a calorie deficit in two ways. First, you will be burning fat during the workout itself, and second, as mentioned above, you will be putting muscle on your body that burns fat twenty-four hours a day—a little furnace within, so to speak, that eats up those excess calories.

WHAT ABOUT FOOD?—SOME CALORIES ARE FATTER THAN OTHERS

Believe it or not, when it comes to eating, it's not *how much* you eat but *what* you eat that counts. Some calories are fatter than others. For example, eight ounces of ice cream will make you a lot fatter than eight ounces of potatoes or eight ounces of lean fish or poultry. Why?

You see, carbohydrates and protein contain only four calories per gram, but fat contains nine calories per gram—more than double that of protein or carbohydrate. But fat is even fatter than that.

When you eat protein or carbohydrates, your body burns up 15 percent to 25 percent of the calories in the digestion process, so that only 75 percent to 85 percent of those calories are available to your body for use as fuel or for fat storage. On the other hand, when you eat a fatty food, only 2 percent to 3 percent of the fat is burned up in the digestion process, and thus 97 percent to 98 percent of that fat is available to your body as fuel or fat storage. In other words, every time you eat a greasy cheeseburger, a big chocolate donut, or a bag of potato chips, you might as well paste them to your thighs, your hips, your stomach, and your buttocks, because that's where they go (these are the favorite storage tanks for fat on women).

Now don't throw this book across the room. There's great news with all of this. You can eat plenty of low-fat foods without getting fat. Baked potatoes, pasta with tomato sauce, low-fat yogurt and frozen yogurt, fresh fruits and vegetables, and low-fat fish and poultry are no problem. You can eat plenty and never go hungry. We (Joyce and Marthe) are constantly snacking—but on the right things.

In Chapter 7 we'll tell you how to pick and choose from your college menu, no matter how bad it is, and how to stock your room (with or without a refrigerator) so that you'll never again be the victim of circumstances. And once you reach your goal, there's something to look forward to. You can eat anything you want one day a week. This too will be explained in Chapter 7.

WHY MOST PEOPLE GAIN BACK MORE WEIGHT THAN THEY LOST WHEN THEY RESORT TO LIQUID AND/OR STARVATION DIETS

There are two problems with liquid diets. 1) The body wants chewable food, not once a day, as is allowed on most liquid diets, but three to five times a day. 2) If you deprive your body of the natural right to chew, it will lie in wait for the day when the liquid diet is over and you are off guard. For example, if you have a fight with your boyfriend, or you flunk an exam, or your parents are giving you a hard time, your body will take over and for some seemingly strange reason you won't be able to stop eating. And you will eat and eat and eat until your body believes that it has experienced the chewing of any and every food it has missed—including all of the fatty foods that make you gain weight. What makes this impulse even worse is, most liquid diets keep your calorie intake so low that your body is near its starvation level. This doubles your drive to binge the moment your mind is relaxed. If you have any doubt about this, just read the literature on the success rate of liquid diets. Most people who go on them gain back the weight they lost in less than a year's time—with some extra weight in the bargain.

You can't win by starving the body either, even if you are starving it with solid foods. It will beat you every time, because it is a survival system. Although your mind is powerful, and you can temporarily use it to starve yourself by sheer willpower, the day will come when your body will take over, and when it does it will make sure it gets back more than it lost, in order to prepare for the next time you might try to deprive it.

It makes me sick to hear people brag, "I didn't eat a thing all day," or, "I only eat one meal a day," because I know that doing this will only make them fatter in the long run. Why? Not only because they will have a strong urge to binge at the end of the day, but when you cut your calories below 1,000, your metabolism slows down in order to prevent what it perceives as a threat to your life. The survival system takes over, and your body begins burning the meager calories you put into it at a slower rate, in the hope of stretching them out in order to live longer. So these foolish people are suffering for nothing. They could be eating low-fat, high-energy foods three to five times during the day, and losing more weight—and not suffering at all!

The bottom line is: there are no short cuts. If you want to lose weight and keep it off, you have to do it by eating plenty of low-fat, nutritious, filling, chewable foods so that your metabolism will not slow down, and your body will not take over and force you to eat until you gain all the weight you so painfully lost—and then some.

HOW LONG WILL IT TAKE TO SEE RESULTS?

You will begin to see definition forming in your upper back and shoulder area in about ten days. In three weeks, your entire body will begin to feel harder, and you will see your biceps and triceps beginning to take shape. In four weeks you will notice that your stomach has become flatter. In five to six weeks, your buttocks will be reduced and will be higher, and your thighs will be firmer and will have definition. In ten weeks, you'll look and feel in shape. You'll no longer be obsessed with your weight because you'll love what you see in the mirror. (If you are more than fifteen pounds overweight, allow an extra week for each pound and a half over.)

FORGET THE SCALE—LOOK IN THE MIRROR

If you are up to fifteen pounds overweight, you will lose weight at a rate of about one half to two pounds a week. But don't become preoccupied with the scale. It's what you see in the mirror that counts. Scale weight varies as your water weight fluctuates due to menstruation and sodium intake. It also changes as you build muscle and eliminate body fat.

Muscle weighs more than fat but takes up less space. For this reason, as you follow this program, you will soon fit into a smaller size jeans—but your scale weight may not go down as much as you had hoped. Why is this so? Think of muscle as lead and fat as feathers. When you lose five pounds of fat you've created muscle where fat used to be, so you've added three pounds of muscle, which takes up less space than the fat (hence the smaller size jeans), but is dense, and thus weighs more. So even though you lost five pounds of fat, your scale weight will only go down by two pounds. But who cares. If you look in the mirror, you can see that you look as if you lost ten pounds!

YOU MAY NOT HAVE TO LOSE AS MUCH WEIGHT AS YOU THINK!

So stop worrying about the scale. In time, if you are fifteen pounds overweight, of course you will lose weight. But you may not have to lose the full fifteen pounds you thought you had to lose, because now that you will have muscle, your body composition will have changed. You will probably find that if you follow this workout, you will have to lose five pounds less than you thought you had to lose. Let the mirror be your guide.

WHAT ABOUT CELLULITE?

Cellulite is really just bunched-up fat that looks like dimples. It resembles the surface of an orange peel. Some people are more genetically inclined to it than others, so you may see some on your body even now. But no matter. This workout will make quick work of getting rid of it— once and for all. As you exercise, and follow the low-fat eating plan, you will burn away the bunched-up fat and place a toned muscle under your skin. Your body will be smooth, shapely, and appealing. It's that simple.

THIS PROGRAM IS FOR YOU EVEN IF YOU ARE NOT OVERWEIGHT!

Even if you are not overweight, you can always improve your body shape. The only way to perfect every part of your body—to shape perfectly formed thighs, high, tight buttocks, well-defined, beautiful shoulders, a V-shaped back that helps the waist look smaller, curvaceous arms, and a flat, defined stomach with a steel girdle of muscle—is to work with weights the right way. That way is presented in this book.

It's not good enough to just be able to say, "I'm not overweight." What you need to be able to say is, "I'm in shape." In addition, if you start working out now, you will be able to head off possible weight problems in the future. So think of this program as an insurance policy against getting fat or getting out of shape.

If you're not overweight, but want to get into perfect shape, allow ten weeks to get to your perfect body.

YOUR BODY WILL CONTINUE TO IMPROVE

What happens after ten weeks? As you continue to do the workout, and follow the maintenance eating plan (now you get to eat anything you want all day long, once a week), your body will continue to look better and better as your muscles become "seasoned"—more and more shapely, more and more defined—and harder and harder, sexier and sexier.

YOU GET MORE THAN A BEAUTIFUL BODY

In addition to all of the above, this program will help you to improve your concentration and your ability to organize yourself, and perhaps even your grades. A simple thing like incorporating a daily twenty-minute workout into your busy day, and the self-discipline it takes to follow through on it in spite of what's going on around you, will quickly carry over to other areas. You'll find that, mysteriously, when it comes to studies, you are putting first things first more often than you are used to—college work before social life—in order to maintain your grade point average. To your own amazement, you may find yourself saying, "I'll let you know later if I can go out. It depends on whether or not I've finished ..."

You'll notice another carryover in the area of concentration. Since working out requires that you focus your full attention on the exercises at hand, when you're trying to study you will find that your mind does not wander away as often as it used to.

Finally, working out is a great relief from college stress. Instead of skipping a workout the night before an exam, I (Marthe) find myself looking forward to it as an outlet to vent frustration, because after I've exercised I feel much more calm about studying. You let go of some tension with each repetition. You'll see what I mean once you start working out.

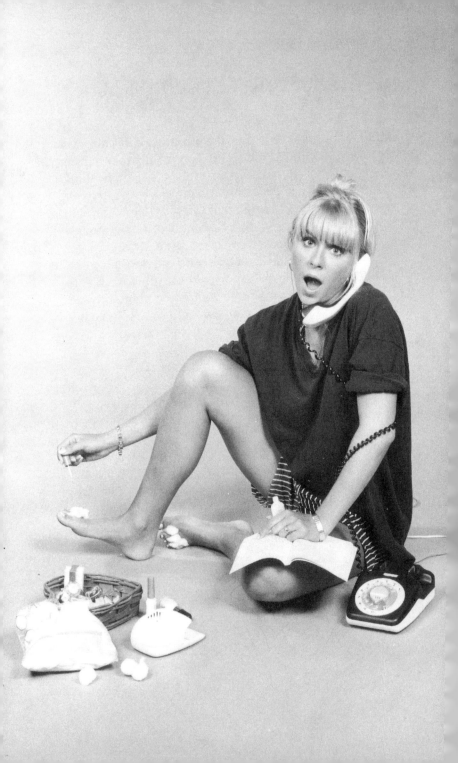

2

FYI (FOR YOUR INFORMATION)

In order to speed through your workout without having to stop and review, take the time to read this chapter before you start. Later, if you forget something you read here, you can go back and review, but chances are you won't have to do that because the information is simple and will stay in your mind after you read it once.

EXERCISE

The following exercise terms will be used time and again in chapters 3 through 5.

An **exercise** is the specific body-shaping movement being performed. For example, the incline flye is a chest exercise.

A **repetition** or **rep** is a complete movement of a given exercise, from starting point to midpoint and back to starting point again. For example, one repetition of the incline flye involves raising the arms straight up with a dumbbell held in each hand, extending the arms outward in an arc-like movement, and returning the arms to the straight-up position.

A **set** is a designated number of repetitions to be performed without resting. In this workout, you will do sets of ten repetitions for all upper body and calf exercises, sets of twelve to fifteen repetitions for all thigh exercises, and sets of fifteen to twenty-five repetitions for all hip-buttocks and abdominal exercises.

A **rest** is a brief pause between sets. Resting allows the working muscle time to recuperate so that it can function at optimum capacity. This is a very intense workout. You will only be allowed to rest after you have completed a giant set consisting of three exercises for a body part.

A **giant set** is the performance of three exercises without taking a rest. In this workout, you will giant-set your entire routine for each body part. For example, in your chest routine, you will do ten repetitions each of the incline press, the pec squeeze, and the incline flye before you take a fifteen-second rest. Then you will repeat the giant set twice more before moving to your shoulder routine, which you will also giant-set. More about this in Chapter 3.

Intensity is the degree of difficulty of the exercise program—specifically, the amount of energy or effort it takes to perform the program. The higher the intensity, the more you will get out of it. Intensity can be increased by shortening rest periods or eliminating them, and by flexing and applying **dynamic tension** (continual pressure). This workout incorporates both shortened rests and continual pressure so that maximum intensity is achieved.

A **routine** is the total amount of exercises performed for a given body part. For example, in this workout, your chest routine consists of three exercises, the incline press, the pec squeeze, and the incline flye.

A **workout** is the combination of all exercises done on a given day. For example, in this program your upper body workout consists of the following routines: chest, shoulders, biceps, triceps, and back. The term "workout" can also be applied to your overall workout—the total combination of exercises on all workout days.

A **split routine** is the exercising of specified body parts on different days. There are two- and three-day split routines. This workout is a two-day split routine. The split routine is used because it has been discovered that in order to achieve optimum growth and development, most muscles need a minimum of forty-eight hours to rest before being challenged again. In other words, it would not be a good idea to exercise your chest, shoulders, biceps, triceps, and back two days in a row. Notice that in this workout you exercise thighs, hip-buttocks, abdominals, and calves the day after you exercise the upper body. In this way, you give your upper body muscles a day to rest, but at the same time you do not waste time because you exercise the other half of your body.

You will use **muscle isolation** in this workout, a method of exercising a body part completely and independently of other body parts. This method insures that you provide each body part with enough uninterrupted work so that the muscle is forced to grow and develop. As mentioned before, systems such as circuit training, where one or two sets are performed for a body part, *cannot* reshape muscle. Such systems are better than nothing, of course, because they stimulate the muscle and burn some calories, but they cannot reshape the body.

The following group of expressions will be encountered time and again in the exercise instructions.

To **flex** the muscle is to contract or squeeze together

the fibers of the muscle. For example, when performing the simultaneous biceps curl, the biceps are contracted when you bend your arms to the highest point. At this point, your biceps muscles bulge. When we say flex your muscle as hard as possible in the exercise instructions, we mean consciously squeeze or contract the muscle as intensely as you can, over and above the normal bending or flexing position the muscle will be in at that point.

To **stretch** the muscle is to elongate the muscle fibers and the muscle. For example, when performing the biceps simultaneous curl, the biceps muscles are stretched when you bring your arms down to their lowest position. At this point your biceps muscles seem to flatten out. When we say apply pressure or tension on the stretch part of the exercise, we mean exert dynamic tension (see below).

You use **dynamic tension** when you exert force on your muscle as it is being stretched or elongated. For example, dynamic tension is applied to your chest muscles when you are performing the incline flye if you exert pressure on your working muscle as you extend your arms outward, as the muscle stretches.

If you continually flex and use dynamic tension as you are exercising, you will be using the principle of **continual pressure**, and will be increasing the intensity of the workout. This constant exertion of force on the working muscle will increase your progress. Continual contraction on the flexing part of the movement and constant tension on the stretching part of the movement provide a self-created force and can be more effective than the adding of heavier weights. In this workout, rather than have you progress to very heavy weights, you will use five-pound dumbbells and instead exert more and more pressure as you become stronger and stronger.

You will be using **free weights**, specifically, dumbbells, with this workout, as opposed to machines.

A **dumbbell** is a short metal bar with a weight on each end. Dumbbells are designed to be held in each hand.

ANATOMY

After working out for about two weeks, you will begin to see changes taking place in your body. Definition will begin to appear, and that definition will continue to increase each week as you continue to work out. In about a month, you'll notice muscle density, which will also increase as you go along. Finally, in three months, you'll notice a great change in your body symmetry—your body will be more balanced, more pleasing to the eye.

Your muscles have **definition** when you can see a fully delineated or defined muscle due to the absence of surrounding body fat. The high repetition–continual pressure aspect of this workout, coupled with the low-fat diet, will result in excellent muscle definition.

Your muscles will have **density**, or hardness or firmness, as a result of using continual pressure when working out.

You have overall **symmetry** when you have aesthetic balance and proportion in the muscles of your body. This workout is designed to help you create near-perfect symmetry for your body. (There is no such thing as perfect symmetry on the human body.)

If you want near-perfect symmetry, it's a good idea to do the entire workout, and not just select body parts that you think need work.

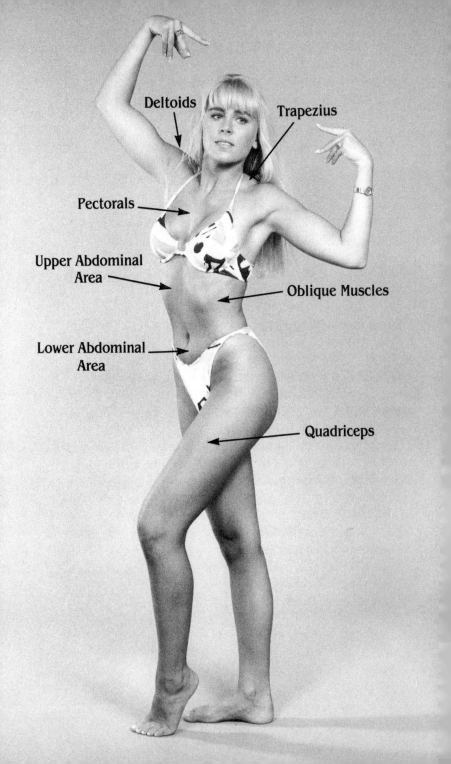

Deltoids

Trapezius

Pectorals

Upper Abdominal
Area

Oblique Muscles

Lower Abdominal
Area

Quadriceps

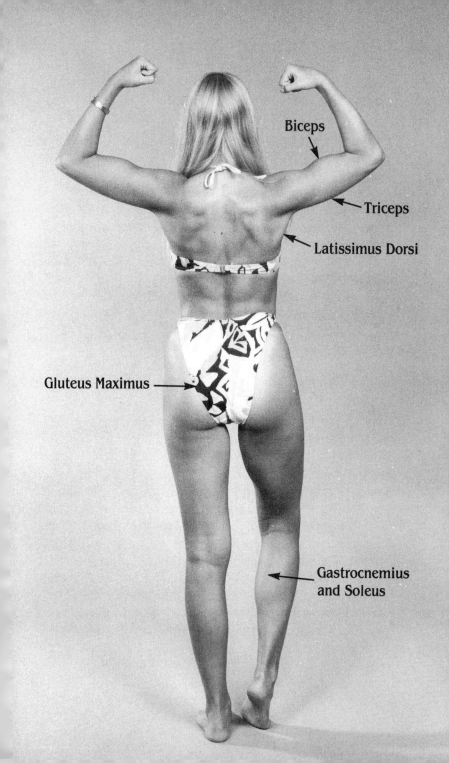

Biceps

Triceps

Latissimus Dorsi

Gluteus Maximus

Gastrocnemius
and Soleus

KNOW YOUR MUSCLES!

Before you start the workout, take a look at the anatomy photographs, and use them to locate the muscles listed below on your own body. Read each muscle description and think of your own muscle. Then, as you work out, continually think of the working muscle as you move. Whenever possible, touch the working muscle with your free hand. Feel it flexing and stretching. "Tell" the working muscle to grow and to be shaped into its perfect form. Picture this happening as you work.

The muscle descriptions are listed in the order that they appear in the workout.

Chest
(Pectoralis Major, Pectorals, or "Pecs")

The **pectoralis major** is a two-headed, fan-shaped muscle that lies across the front of the upper chest. The clavicular head that is the smallest of the two heads forms the upper pectoral area, while the larger sternal head forms the lower pectoral area. The pectoralis muscles originate at the collarbone and run along the breastbone to the cartilage connecting the upper ribs to the breastbone. These muscles are covered by the fatty tissue known as breasts. Breast size can increase only by adding fat to that area; however, breast size can appear to increase and can appear to be uplifted if the pectoral muscles are well developed. In addition, well-developed pectoral muscles give the chest muscles definition, in other words, "cleavage."

Shoulder
(Deltoids)

The **deltoid** is a triangular muscle that resembles an inverted version of the Greek letter delta. It has three parts that can function independently or as a group: the anterior (front deltoid), the medial (middle or side deltoid), and the posterior (rear deltoid).

The entire deltoid muscle originates in the upper area of the shoulder blade, where it joins the collarbone. The three parts of the muscle weave together and are attached on the bone of the upper arm. One angle drapes over the shoulder area, another points down the arm, weaving around the front of that arm, and the third drapes down the back of the arm.

The anterior deltoid works with the pectoral muscles to lift the arm and to move it forward. The medial deltoid helps to lift the arm sideways; and the posterior deltoid works in conjunction with the latissimus dorsi to extend the arm backward.

Biceps

The **biceps** is a two-headed muscle with one short head and one longer head. Both heads originate on the cavity of the shoulder blade where the upper arm bone inserts into the shoulder. The two heads join to form a "hump" about one third down the arm. The other end of the biceps muscle is attached to the bones of the forearm by one connecting tendon.

The biceps muscle works to twist the hand and to flex the arm. The simultaneous curl, the hammer curl, and the concentration curl challenge the biceps muscle.

Triceps

The **triceps** muscle, located just opposite the biceps muscle, consists of three heads. One of the heads attaches to the shoulder blade, while the other two originate from the back side of the upper arm and insert at the elbow.

The longer head of the triceps muscle functions to pull the arm back once it has been moved away from the body, while the other two heads, in conjunction with the longer head, work to extend the arm and the forearm.

Back
(Latissimus Dorsi and Trapezius)

The **latissimus dorsi** muscles originate along the spinal column in the middle of the back, travel upward and sideways to the shoulders, and insert in the front of the upper arm.

The latissimus dorsi are the muscles that help to give the back its V shape or its width. Well-developed "lats" can help your waist to appear smaller. These muscles work to pull the shoulders back and downward and the arm toward the body.

The **trapezius** is a triangular muscle that originates along the spine and runs from the back of the neck to the middle of the back. The upper fibers of the trapezius are attached to the collarbone and show up in the neck-shoulder area.

The upper trapezius muscles function to shrug the shoulders and pull the head back, while the lower part of the muscle group helps to support the shoulder blade when the arm is raised in an above-the-head position.

Thighs
(Quadriceps and Biceps Femoris—Hamstrings)

The **quadriceps**, or front thigh muscle, extends the leg from the bent position. It consists of four muscles: the rectus femoris and the vasti (there are three vasti muscles altogether). The rectus femoris originates on a ridge on the front of the hip bone, while the three vasti muscles originate in various parts of the thigh bone. These muscles join at the kneecap.

The back thigh is composed of the **biceps femoris** and semimembranosus and semitendinosus muscles. Together, this muscle group is called the **hamstrings**.

The biceps femoris is a two-headed muscle that, in co-operation with the semimembranosus and semitendinosus muscles, works to bend the knee. These muscles originate in the bony area of the pelvis and end along the back knee joint.

Hips and Buttocks
(Gluteus Maximus, Gluteus Medius, and Gluteus Minimus)

The largest of the gluetus muscles, the **gluteus maximus**, originates from the iliac crest of the thigh bone and runs down to the tailbone. It extends and rotates the thigh when extreme force is needed, as in running or climbing.

The **gluteus medius** is located just beneath the gluteus maximus. It raises the leg out to the side and balances the hips as weight is transferred from one foot to the other.

The **gluteus minimus** originates on the iliac crest of the hip bone, and performs the same function as the gluteus medius.

Abdominals
(Rectus Abdominis, External Obliques, and Internal Obliques)

The **rectus abdominis** is an elongated, segmented muscle that pulls the torso or upper body toward the lower body when sitting up from a lying-down position. The "abs" originate from the fifth, sixth, and seventh ribs and run vertically up and down across the abdominal wall.

Although the rectus abdominis is actually one long muscle, it is always discussed in the plural because of its segmented nature and the division into upper and lower sections for purposes of exercise.

The **external oblique** muscles originate at the side of the lower ribs and run diagonally to the rectus abdominis. They are attached to the sheath of fibrous tissue that surrounds the rectus abdominis. These muscles work with other muscles to rotate and flex the torso.

The **internal oblique** muscles lie beneath the external obliques, and run at right angles to them. It is this angle that forms the shape of the waistline and that determines its size.

Calves
(Gastrocnemius and Soleus Muscles)

The **gastrocnemius** is a two-headed muscle that connects in the middle of the lower leg and ties in with the Achilles tendon. The point where the two muscles are tied together forms the calf muscle.

The gastrocnemius helps to bend the knee and flex the foot downward. It works in opposition to the extensor muscles of the lower leg, which pull the foot upward.

The **soleus** muscle originates on the back of the tibia

and head of the fibula bones. It lies just underneath the gastrocnemius muscle, but does not pass the knee joint. For this reason, the muscle can flex the foot downward, but cannot help to bend the knee.

In this workout you will be using all of the muscles mentioned above, some of which have been previously neglected. The day after your first workout, you will be reminded that these muscles exist!

EXPECT SOME SORENESS

Even if you follow the break-in-gently plan, you can expect a fair amount of soreness the day after you work out. This is normal, because your muscles are being challenged in a way that they have never been challenged before.

Muscles become sore because of the eccentric contraction of the muscles (the part of the exercise where you lower, rather than raise, the weight). When you lower the weight, the muscle fibers are challenged to the maximum because they are lengthening while at the same time they are attempting to contract. The end result is minute tears in the muscle tissue itself. It is these tears that cause the soreness. In addition, a small amount of fluid is retained in the surrounding tissues, adding to the discomfort and the feeling of soreness.

Another type of muscle soreness may occur while you are performing your workout. If you are working harder than you've worked before, and are at your capacity, your muscle will experience a lack of oxygen and begin to ache. A few seconds after you stop exercising, however, the ache will go away. Such aches are harmless, and are in fact a good sign. They mean that you are giving it all you've got!

WORK THROUGH THE SORENESS

No matter what you do, don't take a day off from working out just because you are sore. Instead, work through the soreness. The workout itself will act as a massage and will help you to feel better as you stimulate your stiff muscles with a fresh circulation of blood.

CAN YOU BECOME INJURED
WITH THIS WORKOUT?

You can become injured doing anything, even walking down the stairs—if you are not careful! But since you will be using relatively light weights in this workout, and will be following the exercise instructions and photographs, your chance of injury will be very slim.

How can you tell if you are injured? How will you know that it is not just soreness? It's easy. Soreness is a pain on a much lower level. It comes after about twenty-four to forty-eight hours of working out, and disappears after a while (anywhere from three days to a week, depending upon the extent of the soreness). The pain that comes from injury comes immediately, is usually sharp and abrupt, and usually makes it impossible for you to continue working out with any kind of ease. Such pain does not gradually disappear, but rather increases unless treated.

An example of an injury is a muscular tear. When you tear a muscle, you feel an incapacitating pain. This can occur if you jerk a weight too quickly. Other common injuries are tendon and ligament injuries. All of these injuries require medical attention (braces, taping, pain-relief medication, and so on). If you think you are injured, you probably are. Don't take a chance. Check with your doctor immediately.

WORK AROUND INJURIES

If you experience an injury, not just in weight training, which as discussed above is very unlikely, but in any other area (say, for example, you have a skiing accident and you break your leg), don't completely stop working out. Exercise those body parts that are not involved in the injury. For example, if you break a leg, you can still exercise your chest, shoulders, biceps, triceps, back, and abdominals, and even to some extent your hip-buttocks area.

In time, your doctor may encourage you to exercise the injured area with light weights. Check with him or her regularly, because injuries can heal faster with light supervised workouts.

The point is, if you are injured, the last thing you should do is completely vegetate. This would be depressing, and what's more, it's completely unnecessary. If you are injured, with your doctor's approval, "work around it"!

USING YOUR MIND TO SPEED UP YOUR PROGRESS

The most powerful tool you have in succeeding in your workout is your mind. You can use your mind to increase your progress in seven ways.

1. Visualize your future body. Most of us have an idealized image of what we perceive to be the "perfect" body. In fact, many people have a specific model or star in mind. In order to take care of this right now, get a photograph of your idealized model and make a list of the permanent differences between the two of you. You may be shorter or taller, smaller-boned or bigger-boned, younger or older, fairer-skinned or darker-skinned. Make a list. Now face the fact that there are some aspects of this model figure that you can never achieve, nor should you want to. Make an agreement with yourself as to which aspects of the model photo are realistic for you to achieve.

Next, take a full front and back photograph of yourself in a bikini (this will also come in handy later when you are searching for a "before" photo of yourself to prove to others how much progress you have made), and draw over it with magic marker correcting any faults that you perceive in your body—remove fat from your thighs, re-shape your waistline, and so on. Add pretty muscles to your shoulders and arms. Now look at the photograph and imagine yourself evolving into your perfect form.

Next, take a hard look at yourself in the mirror, in the nude. Now mentally re-create your body into its ideal image. Remember to be realistic. You're not going to have narrow hips if you are big-boned, and you're not going to grow five inches if you are short. Imagine *your* best body. Then delight in the fact that your best will be the idealized you—and no one else will be able to duplicate that you either. In fact, take my word for it, once you reach your best—for you—you will no longer be preoccupied with looking like anyone else. Suddenly, in your own eyes, you will be good enough just the way you are, because you will know that you have reached *your* best body. Now picture yourself walking into a party and feeling good about yourself—feeling that you look great—and couldn't hope to look any better, because that's just how you will feel in a matter of time. Then set a realistic time frame to get in shape. (See Chapter 1, and below, for information on a target date.)

2. Tell your muscles to take shape as you exercise. As you move the dumbbells from point A to point B, watch your working muscles, and picture them taking the perfect form you have in mind. Imagine the fat melting away, and the muscle fibers increasing and shaping into tight, well-defined, sensuous muscle. In fact, go a step further than that. Actually tell your muscles to grow into their perfect form, and order the fat to go away with each repetition. Of course you're not always going to remember to, or even feel like doing this, but do it whenever you think of it and are in the mood, because by linking your mind into full cooperation with your body, you can increase your progress as much as 50 percent. Athletes do it all the time. Bodybuilders, boxers, basketball players, dancers, marathon runners, and a host of others regularly use mind-body techniques in order to make every moment of training count.

3. Set a goal and let your mind lead your body to it. The mind is like a homing torpedo. If you give it a realistic goal, it will zigzag its way around obstacles in order to lead you to the goal.

When you come to think of it, your mind does this all the time for you when it comes to term papers and exams. As you go through your semester, you are aware that at certain intervals term papers are due and exams are scheduled. These events, whether or not you officially label them as such, are goals. Somehow the paper gets handed in on the due date, and the exam gets taken with some success on exam day. Why?

Your unconscious mind registered the information and realized that it had a goal that must be achieved by a certain date. So after your body fought you a hundred times when you insisted upon lying around watching television, your mind forced your body to rise from the couch and zigzag around the obstacle to achieve the goal—the preparation for the exam, or the writing of the term paper—on target date.

When you cooperate with your mind, and join forces with it by actively willing to achieve your goal on target date, your mind can zigzag you to your goal that much more efficiently. For example, with the workout, if you set a target date and then use the preconditioning techniques below, your mind cooperates that much more in getting you to your goal. For example, to your probable amazement, there will be times when you had every intention of skipping a workout, but then, for some strange reason, you will pick up the dumbbells and start moving. Other times you will be ready to eat some fat-filled food, and then suddenly you'll decide not to. This will be your unconscious mind behaving like a homing torpedo, zigzagging you around obstacles to reach your goal.

4. Precondition yourself to do your workout and follow the low-fat eating plan. In order to help your unconscious mind do its work, it's a good idea to think ahead and precondition your mind to overcome obstacles that would hinder your progress. For example, think ahead of the following scenario. You usually work out first thing in the morning, but when the alarm rings, you don't want to get up because you were out late last night. You wake up and you tell yourself, "I can't do it. I don't need this. I'm too tired," and you are about to turn over in your bed after pressing the snooze button.

Picture this scene ahead of time, and tell yourself when that happens, with the very thought, "I'm too tired," you will experience a sudden burst of energy, jump out of bed, and without further negotiation pick up the dumbbells and start working out, knowing that in twenty minutes it will all be over, and that later in the day when you otherwise would be ready to start berating yourself for having missed a workout, you will rejoice when you realize that, in fact, you did work out!

You can do the same thing with food situations. Picture yourself about to indulge in a fatty food such as a donut or a greasy hamburger, and then imagine yourself suddenly getting a nauseous feeling and pushing it away, and instead reaching for a low-fat food such as a big bowl of strawberries, a container of yogurt, or a baked potato.

Preconditioning works because it is your way of agreeing with yourself ahead of time that you really do want to achieve the goal. In a sense, preconditioning is a coming together of the conflicting aspects of your whole being. It's like joining forces with yourself.

5. Help yourself with discipline. In order to help yourself to achieve your goal, it is important to set a daily time for working out, and then do it every day at that time. The morning is the best time, but if that isn't possible, do it in the afternoons or evening—but for discipline's sake, do it the same time every day. If you can't manage that, set a specific time each day and write it into your schedule the way you would a class, and then, come hell or high water, do it! The key is you must schedule your workout into your daily plan, and then keep your appointment with yourself and do that workout the same way you would keep an appointment with any other important person.

6. Think of the prize and compare it to the price. When you are tempted to skip a workout, or to abandon your good eating habits, think of the price you are paying (twenty minutes six days a week and never-go-hungry, low-fat eating) and compare it with the prize. And what is that prize?

Freedom from the mental torture that drains your psychological and even physical energy, the voice that says, "You're fat and are getting fatter every day. You're out of control. There's nothing you can do about it. Nobody will want to go out with you. You are a hopeless case." Once you begin the workout and the eating plan and you no longer negotiate the issue, you will be free, once and for all, of the mental torment because you will know that finally you are in control of your body. You will realize that although it won't happen overnight, it will happen, and you will have the body of your dreams. But what's more important, you will know that you are no longer growing fatter and more out of shape every day—and that you will never again be in that position.

Once you feel in control of your body, your self-confidence in general will increase, because you will realize that the same way you were able to exert self-discipline in a previously unconquerable area, the body, you will be able to control other areas where you used to allow yourself to be victimized, such as relationships, school matters, work, and later, career. In fact, there will be a carryover effect in facing any challenge that comes your way, because you will know that you can take control of a situation, and with calm action effect change.

7. When you slip up, instead of badmouthing yourself, forgive yourself and go on from there! No matter how determined you are, there will be times when you just blow it. So what. You're only human. Instead of letting negative verbalizations rule the day (if you're not careful, you'll start believing them), and instead of letting that voice in your head go on and on with statements such as "You're a lazy pig. You'll never keep up with this. What made you dream you could do it—you never follow through with anything," stop the music right there.

Play a different tune. Answer yourself back with such statements as, "Big deal. I did a very natural thing. I gave in to my urge to relax and/or to eat. But that was a temporary lapse. I am in control. I can decide to get on track again, and I'm going to do it right now, and even if I do slip again and again, it's the big picture that counts. As long as I don't give up, in time I'll reach my goal—and soon there will be fewer and fewer slips. It's all up to me. I decide whether I will achieve this goal or not."

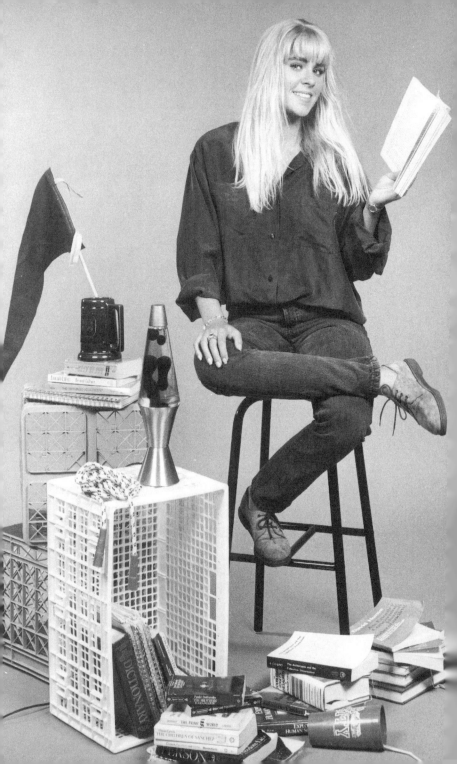

3

HOW TO DO THE COLLEGE DORM WORKOUT

This workout is very simple to perform. You do the weight workout in your dorm with a pair of five-pound dumbbells—standing, sitting on the bed or a chair, and lying on the floor. If you choose Plan A, you do the straight aerobic part of the workout anywhere—in your dorm with a jump rope; outside, walking or running; or in the school gym on the exercise bike, the stair-stepper, or any other aerobic machine.

First we'll explain how to do the weight workout, and then we'll talk about workout schedules.

WORKOUT DAY ONE: UPPER BODY

On workout day one, you will exercise chest, shoulders, biceps, triceps, and back, in that order. Here is your exercise list and repetition and set guide.

Chest

Incline press
Pec squeeze
Incline flye

Shoulders

Side lateral
Front lateral
Bent lateral

Biceps

Simultaneous curl
Hammer curl
Concentration curl

Triceps

One-arm extension
Kickback
Cross-face extension

Back

Reverse bent-dumbbell row
Upright row
Seated back lateral

Upper Body Routine

REPETITIONS: Ten repetitions for each set of each exercise. Since you will be doing ten repetitions for each of three separate exercises before you take a rest, you will be doing thirty repetitions per giant set.

SETS: Three giant sets for each exercise.

EXPLANATION OF GIANT SET: This entire workout is based upon the giant set. This means you do your first set of all three of the exercises in your routine for a given body part before you take a fifteen-second rest. Then you do your second set of all three exercises for that body part before you take another fifteen-second rest. Finally, you do your third and last set of all three exercises for that body part. Then you rest fifteen seconds and move to the next body part and work in the same manner.

Chest Routine

Chest Routine Sample

Let's talk about the chest routine first. (Each of the upper body routines is done exactly in this manner.)

SET 1: To do the first exercise, the incline press, you sit in a chair, holding the dumbbells and leaning back in the chair, and you raise the dumbbells until your arms are fully extended and your elbows are nearly locked, then you return to start position (see photos on page 73). You do ten repetitions of the incline press, and without resting, you do your second chest exercise, the pec squeeze, by bringing your arms in and away from your chest (see photos on page 75). You do ten repetitions of this exercise without resting, and you do your final chest exercise, the incline flye, by sitting in the chair and leaning back, extending your arms upward and then moving your arms outward in an arc-like position, and back to the arms extended upward position. You do ten repetitions of this exercise, and then you rest for fifteen seconds.

SET 2: Repeat the entire sequence as above. Rest fifteen seconds.

SET 3: Repeat the entire sequence for the last time. Then rest fifteen seconds and begin your next body part, the shoulder routine.

Shoulder Routine

Shoulder Routine Sample

You will work in exactly the same manner as above, giant-setting your entire shoulder routine.

SET 1:   You do your first set of ten repetitions for the first shoulder exercise, the side lateral, extending your arms out and in, and without resting you do ten repetitions of the next shoulder exercise, the front lateral, raising your arms out in front of you and down, and, again without resting, you do ten repetitions of the third shoulder exercise, the bent lateral, bending down and extending your arms out to the sides and back in (see pages 79–83 for photographs). Then you will rest fifteen seconds.

SET 2:   Repeat the entire sequence. Rest fifteen seconds.

SET 3:   Repeat the sequence for your third and final time. Then rest fifteen seconds and move to your next body part, your biceps routine.

You will then do your biceps, triceps, and back routines in exactly the same manner as above.

It's So Simple and It Really Moves Fast

It's so simple, and it moves so fast, and there's really so little to remember. For your entire upper body workout, all you do is continue to do your ten repetitions of each of three exercises for a given body part without resting until you've done one giant set, consisting of a grand total of thirty repetitions, ten distinct repetitions for each of three separate exercises for that body part, then rest fifteen seconds and repeat the sequence, then rest fifteen seconds and repeat the sequence a third and final time, for a grand total of three giant sets comprised of three exercises per body part.

See how easy it is. And the best part of all of this is that the exercises have been carefully designed so you don't often have to jump up and move all over the place to change position for the next exercise. You will quickly see this as you begin following the exercise photographs and instructions.

You will be reminded to flex and apply continual tension to your working muscle in the exercise instructions, and just in case you forget, you will be reminded of how many repetitions to do, and when to stop and take your big fifteen-second rest.

WORKOUT DAY TWO: LOWER BODY

Your lower body workout is exactly the same *except* you will be doing a different number of repetitions for certain body parts. Your lower body workout will cover thighs, which require twelve to fifteen repetitions per exercise; hip-buttocks, which require fifteen to twenty-five repetitions per exercise; abdominals, which require fifteen to twenty-five repetitions per exercise; and calves, which require ten repetitions per exercise.

Don't worry that you will get confused about how many repetitions. The instructions are clear, and after a very short while you'll simply say to yourself, "Thighs—twelve to fifteen," or "Hip-Buttocks and Abs, fifteen to twenty-five," and so on. But to help you etch the number of reps for each body part in your mind, you will be reminded time and again in the exercise instructions.

Here is your lower body exercise list. Your repetition and set guide is listed separately for each lower body part.

Thighs

Squat
Lunge
Leg extension

Hip-Buttocks

Feather kick-up
One-legged butt lift
Scissors

Abdominals

Bent-knee sit-up (or crunch)
Knee-in (or reverse crunch)
Oblique crunch

Calves

Seated straight-toe raise
Seated angled-out toe raise
Seated angled-in toe raise

Thigh Routine

THIGH REPETITIONS: Twelve to fifteen repetitions for each set of each exercise. Since you will be doing twelve to fifteen repetitions for each of three separate exercises before you take a rest, you will be doing thirty-six to forty-five repetitions per giant set.

SETS: Three giant sets for each exercise.

Thigh Routine Sample

You will perform your thigh routine exactly the same way you performed each body part of your upper body routine, in giant sets, only instead of doing ten repetitions for each exercise in a giant set, you will do twelve to fifteen reps. Let's go through it together.

SET 1: You will do your first set of twelve to fifteen repetitions of the squat, and without resting, you will do your first set of twelve to fifteen repetitions of the lunge, and again without resting, you will do your first set of twelve to fifteen repetitions of the leg extension. Then you will rest fifteen seconds.

SET 2: Repeat the sequence exactly as above and then rest fifteen seconds.

SET 3: Repeat the sequence exactly as above. Rest fifteen seconds and move to your hip-buttocks routine.

Hip-Buttocks Routine

The ideal number of repetitions for the hip/buttocks area is fifteen to twenty-five repetitions.

HIP-BUTTOCKS REPETITIONS: Fifteen to twenty-five repetitions for each set of each separate exercise. Since you will be doing fifteen to twenty-five repetitions for each of three separate exercises before you take a rest, you will be doing forty-five to seventy-five repetitions per giant set.

SETS: Three giant sets for each exercise.

Hip-Buttocks Routine Sample

SET 1: You will do your first set of fifteen to twenty-five repetitions of the feather kick-up, and without resting you will do your first set of fifteen to twenty-five repetitions of the one-legged butt lift, and again, without resting, you will do your first set of fifteen to twenty-five repetitions of the scissors. You will then rest fifteen seconds.

SET 2: Repeat the sequence exactly as above and then rest fifteen seconds.

SET 3: Repeat the sequence exactly as above. Rest fifteen seconds, then move to your next body part, the abdominal routine.

Abdominal Routine

Like the hip-buttocks area, the abdominal area responds best to fifteen to twenty-five repetitions, so you will work in exactly the same manner as above.

ABDOMINAL REPETITIONS: Fifteen to twenty-five repetitions for each set of each separate exercise. Since you will be doing fifteen to twenty-five repetitions for each of three separate exercises before you take a rest, you will be doing forty-five to seventy-five repetitions per giant set.

SETS: Three giant sets for each exercise.

There is no need to provide an abdominal example, because you will work in exactly the same manner as for the hip-buttocks routine, doing three giant sets of fifteen to twenty-five repetitions for each exercise.

Calf Routine

The ideal number of repetitions for the calves is ten repetitions.

CALF REPETITIONS: Ten repetitions for each set of each exercise. Since you will be doing ten repetitions for each of three separate exercises before you take a rest, you will be doing thirty repetitions per giant set.

SETS: Three giant sets for each exercise.

There is no need to provide an example for the calf routine, because you will work in the same manner as you did when you exercised all of your upper body parts, doing three sets of ten repetitions for each of the calf exercises, before taking a fifteen-second rest, and then repeating the sequence twice more.

Once you have completed your calf routine, you are finished with your lower body workout.

DECIDING WHETHER TO DO THE MINIMUM OR MAXIMUM AMOUNT OF REPETITIONS WHEN THERE IS A CHOICE

The upper body and calf routines are simple. They leave you no choice. You do ten repetitions for each exercise. End of conversation. But for the thighs, hip-buttocks, and abdominals, you are given a range of reps, because higher repetitions in these areas help to burn more fat and produce more definition.

In the beginning, do the lowest amount required. As you get stronger, you can go to the higher end of the rep range. Later, on certain days when you are tired, you can go back to the lower end of the rep range—for any exercise, at any time. The option is always there for you.

WHAT IF YOU CANNOT MAKE THE MINIMUM NUMBER OF REPS REQUIRED?

If you cannot make the minimum number of reps required, lower your weight. For example, instead of using five-pound dumbbells, use threes or twos—or even ones. It's better to get into the habit of doing all of your reps right from the beginning.

Where weights are not used, such as in the hip-buttocks and abdominal exercises, you may still have trouble making the minimum number of reps in the beginning. In this case, you have no choice but to do fewer for each set. Just do as many reps as you can for each set, perhaps half the required amount until you get stronger. Don't worry.

Before you know it, you'll look back to the time when you couldn't do the reps as a distant memory.

CAN YOU SKIP THE RESTS ALTOGETHER?

Yes. In time, you will get so good at this that you won't want to bother to rest at all. That's fine: as long as you are performing full repetitions, and you remember to flex and use continual tension, you need not rest at all. But realize that in the beginning you will have to take full advantage of your rests because you will be tired.

WHEN DUMBBELLS ARE TOO HEAVY OR LIGHT FOR CERTAIN BODY PARTS

In the beginning, you may find that you can't do certain exercises with the five-pound dumbbells because they are too heavy. You may especially have trouble doing your triceps and shoulder exercises with these dumbbells. If that is the case, get a set of three-pound dumbbells (or lighter) and work up to the five-pound ones.

If you are very strong, you may soon feel that five-pound dumbbells are too light for you—especially for chest, biceps, back, and leg work. Then you will have a choice. You don't have to get heavier dumbbells if you make up for the lightness of the weights by flexing harder and using more dynamic tension; or, instead, you can get a pair of eight- or ten-pound dumbbells.

WHAT ABOUT STRETCHING?

Since you will be using very light weights for this workout, there is no need to stretch. The workout itself serves as its own stretching exercise and warm-up. However, if you wish, you may perform a few repetitions of each exercise without a weight as a warm-up stretch.

BREAKING IN

It's a good idea to break in gently, otherwise you may not be able to get out of bed the next morning, and you may be tempted to quit the workout. So unless you're ready to deal with the extreme soreness, or you have been working out with a similar weight-training program, take your time and break in gently. Here's a good way to do it:

Week 1. Three giant sets of each exercise with no weight.

Week 2. One giant set of each exercise with weight (either three pounds or five pounds—you decide).

Week 3. Two giant sets of each exercise with weight.

Week 4. All three giant sets of each exercise with weight. You are there!

WHAT ABOUT THE AEROBICS?

Your aerobic choices will be discussed in Chapter 6, but in the meantime here's your break-in program for aerobics, based on the assumption that you are not already doing an aerobic activity. (If you are already running, riding an exercise bike, swimming, or doing any other aerobic activity for twenty minutes or more, ignore this schedule and go right to where you are now.)

Week 1. Five minutes a day.
Week 2. Ten minutes a day.
Week 3. Fifteen minutes a day.
Week 4. Twenty minutes a day.

MAKING UP A SCHEDULE

Plan A

Here is how your workout will look:

Sunday	Monday	Tuesday	Wednesday	Thursday	Friday	Saturday
Aerobics	Upper body	Lower body	Aerobics	Upper body	Lower body	Aerobics

Plan B

If you don't like straight aerobics, and would rather do more upper and lower body workouts instead, you may substitute extra upper and lower body workouts for aerobics, because they are in and of themselves aerobic. Here's how your schedule will look if you eliminate the aerobics.

Sunday	Monday	Tuesday	Wednesday	Thursday	Friday	Saturday
Rest	Upper body	Lower body	Upper body	Lower body	Upper body	Lower body

I (Marthe) usually use Plan B or Plan D, because I like working with the weights better than straight aerobics, and because I go fast with the weights and get a full aerobic effect anyway. I like the extra shaping I get with the additional weight workout. But friends of mine have seen equally good results using Plan A, so the choice is yours. It's more important that you enjoy the workout than anything else—because if you hate it, you won't do it. So if you are already doing an aerobic activity that you like, you should use Plan A and incorporate that aerobic activity into your workout.

WHAT IF YOU HAVE TIME TO DO EXTRA WORK?

If you have time to do extra workout sessions, then do Plan B, and add three or more aerobic sessions into your workout. The added aerobics will help you to burn that much more fat. This is Plan C:

Plan C

Sunday	Monday	Tuesday	Wednesday	Thursday	Friday	Saturday
Aerobics	Upper body	Lower body Aerobics	Upper body	Lower body Aerobics	Upper body	Lower body Aerobics

You can do your double-up workouts either one after the other, or space them out. For example, on Tuesday you can do your lower body workout, and then jump rope for twenty minutes, and it's all over, or you can do your lower body workout, go to classes and eat lunch, and then after you study for a few hours, vent your frustration in a twenty-minute aerobic session.

WHAT IF YOU CAN ONLY WORK OUT FOUR DAYS A WEEK?

There's wonderful news. You can still reshape your entire body by working out only four days a week. You will skip the aerobics completely and do your upper and lower body workouts twice each. That will reshape your body and burn plenty of fat. The only thing you will be missing is three days of aerobics, which would have helped you burn additional fat, so if you are trying to lose weight, it will just take you a little longer, but you'll still get there. I usually use Plan D—and switch into Plan B when beach season is approaching.

Plan D—The Bare Minimum

If you can only work out four days a week, here's how your program might look:

Sunday	Monday	Tuesday	Wednesday	Thursday	Friday	Saturday
Rest	Upper body	Lower body	Rest	Upper body	Rest	Lower body

If you are only working out four days a week, it would be ideal if you could space the workout as above, but it isn't necessary to do that. In fact, if your schedule demands it, you can work out four days in a row, and take three days off. Your schedule may then look like this:

Sunday	Monday	Tuesday	Wednesday	Thursday	Friday	Saturday
Lower body	Rest	Rest	Rest	Upper body	Lower body	Upper body

Or like this:

Sunday	Monday	Tuesday	Wednesday	Thursday	Friday	Saturday
Rest	Upper body	Lower body	Upper body	Lower body	Rest	Rest

WHY IS IT OKAY TO SKIP THE AEROBICS BUT NOT THE WEIGHT WORKOUT?

It is very key that you understand this point. If your time is limited, and you have to skip a workout, make sure it is not a weight workout, because it is the weight workout that reshapes your body, has an aerobic effect, and at the same time increases your metabolism (by adding muscle to your body) so that you end up burning more fat twenty-four hours a day.

As mentioned before, and as will be discussed in Chapter 6, straight aerobics are great for burning additional fat and helping to further condition your heart and lungs. They balance out your workout and are fun to do. But if your goal is to get your perfect body, and if it comes down to it that something has to go, let it be the aerobics, and not the weights. We cannot possibly overemphasize this point!

WHAT IF YOU SKIP A WORKOUT?

So what. Just start again. All you have to do is start with whatever half of the body you did not exercise last time. You want to do this because it may be tempting to do the upper body again, even though you did it last time—four days ago. Why? You may hate to do your lower body— thighs, buttocks, stomach, and calves. You must be fair to your body, however, and balance your workout.

What if you end up skipping a lot of workouts, and your average number of weekly weight workouts is two or three? Okay. It's better than nothing, but of course your progress will be slower.

MAKING YOUR OWN SCHEDULE: THE ONLY RULES TO REMEMBER

Now it's time to make up your own schedule. Get a calendar and write your schedule for each day of the week. When constructing your weekly workout, remember the following:

1. Never work your lower body two days in a row, or your upper body two days in a row. Muscles need forty-eight hours to recuperate. The only exception to this rule are the abdominal muscles, which can be exercised every day.
2. Whenever you work out, be sure that you exercise the half of the body that you did *not* exercise last time. For example, say you exercised your upper body on Monday, and then you didn't get to work out for three days. Things came up and now it's Friday. You must work your lower body—the area you did not work the last time you exercised. Doing this will insure that you don't end up with an imbalanced body.
3. Mark your workouts on a calendar. It will make it so much easier for you to remember whether you exercised your upper or lower body the last time.
4. Be sure you get four weight workouts in per week—two upper and two lower. Then you can decide whether you want to do aerobics on the other three days, or add in another upper and lower body workout—or add in both.
5. Straight aerobics can be done anytime, any day, and in any sequence. You can fit them in whenever they are convenient for you.

SET A REALISTIC TARGET DATE
AND MARK IT ON THE CALENDAR

Now that you have evaluated your body, and have read the guidelines as to how quickly you can expect to progress, look at the calendar and set a target date. Don't rush yourself. Be realistic. If you're ten to fifteen pounds overweight and out of shape, think in terms of six to twelve weeks. If you're twenty to twenty-five pounds overweight, think in terms of twelve to twenty-four weeks. Ask yourself how long you need, and go by that. Perhaps you know that you will need a little more time. Rather than rush yourself, set a leisurely target date and aim at that. Maybe you know that you will be able to do it in record time. If so, shorten your time.

Once you decide on a target date, circle it on the calendar and tell yourself to get in shape by that day. Once you circle the date on your calendar, and tell your body to reach your goal by that date, your mind and body will join forces in getting you to your goal on time.

WORK OUT ALONE OR WITH A PARTNER

Whether you decide to work out alone or with a partner will depend upon two things: your personality and partner availability. I (Marthe) like to work out with a partner, because when I do the workout seems to go much faster. Last semester, I used to work out with my roommate, and it seemed as if I wasn't working out at all because we seemed to pick up on each other's energy. Now that she has graduated, and my new roommate's schedule doesn't coincide with mine, I'm working out alone.

At first I thought it was going to be torture, but then to my surprise I found myself looking forward to it. It became a way for me to escape from everything—worries about exams, relationship problems, and life in general. After I focus on my workout for such a short period of time, without anyone else involved, it seems as if I come away not only feeling more relaxed, but with a clearer mind-set.

WHAT IF YOUR ROOM IS VERY SMALL?

Don't worry. This program is designed to be done in even the smallest of rooms—even a typical tiny eight by ten foot room shared with a roommate. You may have to be creative for the floor exercises, and position yourself so that your body can fully stretch out, and you may have to move a chair or two or shove a desk or bed a few inches, but it will work. Where there's a will there's a way, and you will quickly find out that it's well worth the effort.

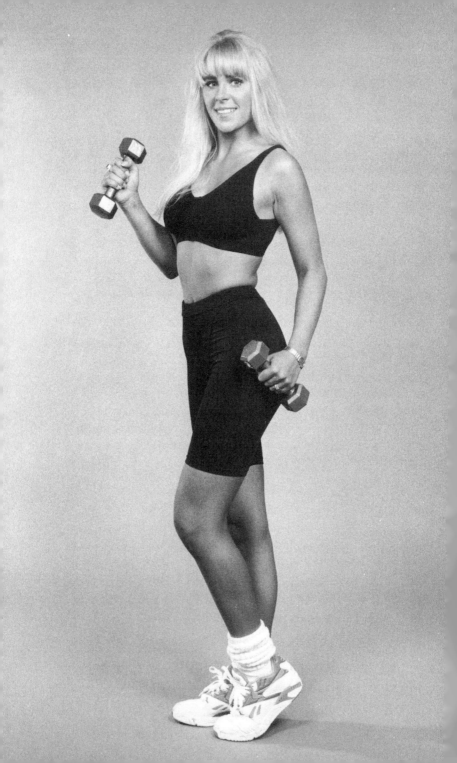

4

UPPER BODY
WORKOUT

Your upper body workout consists of chest, shoulders, biceps and triceps (arms), and back. "But wait a minute," you might be saying. "Why bother to exercise these body parts? All I really care about is my stomach, my rear end, and my thighs."

In order to have a perfectly balanced body, it's necessary to exercise all body parts. Think of how Linda Hamilton would have looked like with strong legs but with thin, jellylike arms and slouching shoulders? And isn't Elle Mc-Pherson's back a major contribution to her beauty? This workout is going to give you the ultimate balanced look of the total-hard body, but only if you do it all—not if you pick and choose.

You will do three exercises for each upper body part—giant-setting all three exercises of each body part, and at the same time flexing and using dynamic tension so that

you can get the most out of the workout. You will rest
fifteen seconds each time you complete a giant set. Follow
the exercise instructions, and you will be reminded when
you can take your fifteen-second rests.

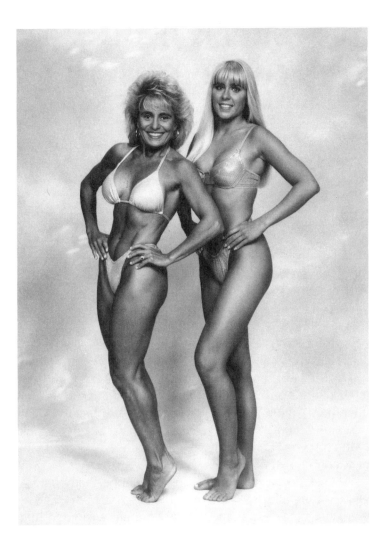

Weights

You will use a five-pound dumbbell for all exercises; however, if you find that five pounds is too heavy for weaker body parts, such as shoulders and triceps, purchase a three-pound dumbbell for these body parts, and then when you get stronger you can use the five-pound dumbbells for everything. (If you only want to purchase one set of dumbbells, and you find that you need the lesser weight of three-pound dumbbells, don't worry that your back, chest, and biceps will suffer from using the lower weight. Just make up for it by flexing and using dynamic tension to the full extent.)

CHEST ROUTINE: INCLINE PRESS, PEC SQUEEZE, INCLINE FLYE

Do three giant sets of ten repetitions of each exercise.

1. Incline Press

This exercise develops and shapes the entire chest (pectoral) area, especially the middle and outer pectorals, and helps to uplift the breasts.

START: Sit in a chair with your buttocks touching the edge of the chair seat and your shoulders touching the back of the chair. Hold a dumbbell in each hand, palms facing upward. The dumbbells should be in a horizontal position as you move them up and down.

MOVE: Squeezing your pectoral muscles as you go, move the dumbbells upward until your arms are fully extended. Without resting, give your pectoral muscles an extra flex, and return to the start position. Without resting, repeat the movement until you have completed your set. Without resting, move to your next chest exercise, the pec squeeze.

TIPS: Be sure to extend your elbows fully downward on each return movement, and to feel the stretch in your chest muscles, and to fully extend your arms

Start

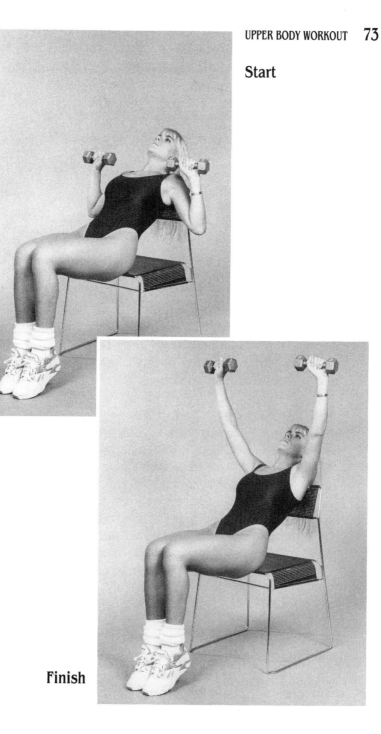

Finish

upward on the up movement. *Do not allow youself to begin taking shortcuts and to begin performing half movements.* This exercise can also be performed on a flat exercise bench, or by placing your shoulders at the edge of a chair or bed.

2. Pec Squeeze

This exercise develops the entire chest (pectoral) muscle, especially the inner area—giving a look of cleavage.

START: Sit at the edge of a chair, holding a dumbbell in each hand. Raise your arms to form two Ls by bending your elbows and extending your arms outward. The dumbbells should be held palms outward, in a vertical position.

MOVE: Simultaneously move your arms toward your chest, squeezing your pectoral muscles all the while, and at the same time maintaining the locked L position of your arms. Continue to move your elbows toward your chest until the dumbbells are touching and your elbows are in line with your breasts. Apply tension to your pectoral muscles on the stretch movement as you return to the start position. Repeat the movement without resting until you have finished your set. Without resting, move to your final chest exercise, the incline flye.

TIPS: Be sure to maintain the L position of your arms throughout the exercise, otherwise you will take

Start

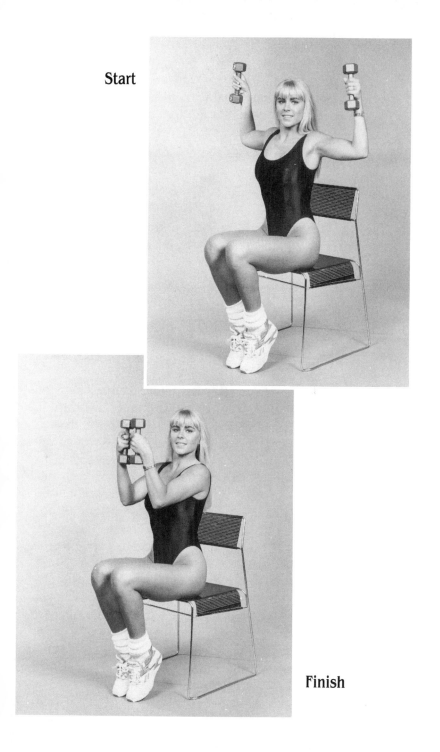

Finish

pressure off your chest muscles. (This exercise is meant to simulate the exercise done on the pec-deck machine found in most gyms.)

3. Incline Flye

This exercise develops, shapes, and defines the entire chest (pectorals) and helps to create cleavage and to give the breasts a firmer, higher look.

START: Place your shoulders against the back of a chair with your feet together, hold a dumbbell in each hand, palms facing each other in the center of your chest, your arms fully extended above you.

MOVE: Applying tension to your pectoral muscles as you go, extend your arms outward and downward in a semicircle until you feel a full stretch in your chest. Flexing your chest muscles as you go, return to the start. Without resting, repeat the movement until you have completed your set. Since you have now completed your first giant set, rest fifteen seconds and then do your second and then third and final giant sets of your chest routine. Then rest fifteen seconds and begin your shoulder routine.

TIPS: Keep your mind on your pectoral muscles as you work. Picture definition and firmness forming. Do not hold your breath. Breathe naturally. This exercise can also be done flat on an exercise bench, or by placing your shoulders at the edge of a chair or bed.

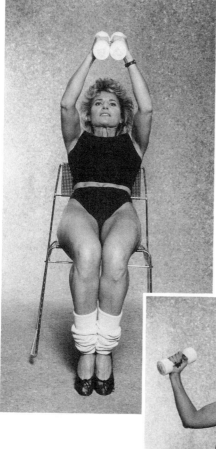

Start

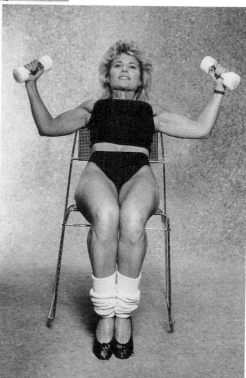

Finish

SHOULDER ROUTINE:
SIDE LATERAL, FRONT LATERAL, BENT LATERAL

Do three giant sets of ten repetitions of each of these exercises.

1. Side Lateral

This exercise develops the side (medial) shoulder (deltoid) muscle.

START: Stand in a natural position with a dumbbell in each hand, palms facing your body, the dumbbells nearly touching at the center of your body.

MOVE: Flexing your shoulder muscles as you go, raise the dumbbells outward, leading with your locked wrists and elbows, until the dumbbells reach ear height. Your elbows will be slightly bent in this position. Keep the tension on your shoulder area and return to the start position. Repeat the movement until you have finished your set. Without resting, move to your next shoulder exercise, the front lateral.

TIPS: Don't rock back and forth as you move the dumbbells. Keep your torso and legs still. The only body parts moving are your arms and shoulders. Keep your mind on your shoulder muscles as you exercise.

Start

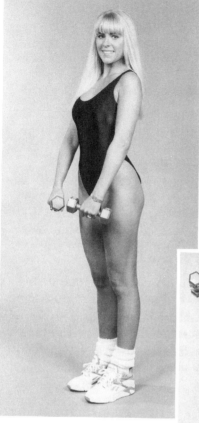

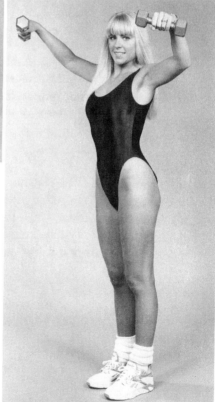

Finish

2. Front Lateral

This exercise develops the front (anterior) shoulder (deltoid) muscle.

START: Stand with your feet in a natural position, holding a dumbbell in each hand. Holding the dumbbells with your palms facing your body, center the dumbbells on each thigh. Your arms should be fully extending downward.

MOVE: Flexing your shoulder muscles, raise one dumbbell until it reaches eye level. Then, as you begin to return that dumbbell to the start position, begin raising the other dumbbell to eye level. Continue this alternate movement until you have completed a full set for each arm. Without resting, move to your last shoulder exercise, the bent lateral.

TIPS: Keep your elbows locked throughout the movement. Don't start wildly swinging the dumbbells up and down. Use steady, deliberate, controlled movements. Keep the pressure and your mind on your working muscle.

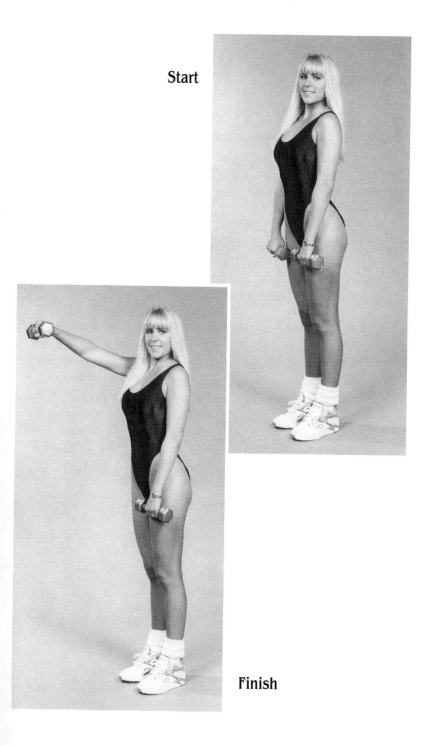

Start

Finish

3. Bent Lateral

This exercise develops the rear (posterior) and side (medial) shoulder (deltoid) muscles.

START: Stand with your feet a natural width apart, with a dumbbell in each hand, palms facing inward. Lean over until your torso is approximately parallel to the floor and let the dumbbells touch each other at the center of your body.

MOVE: Flexing your shoulder muscles as hard as possible, extend your arms outward until they are parallel, or nearly parallel, to the floor. Your elbows should be very slightly bent in this position. Keeping the pressure on your shoulders, return to the start position. Repeat the movement until you have finished your set. Rest fifteen seconds and do your second and then third giant sets of your shoulder routine. Then rest fifteen seconds and begin your biceps routine.

TIPS: Don't rise from the bent-over position as you are exercising. Keep your torso parallel to the floor throughout the movement, or you will take the pressure off your shoulder area and reduce the efficacy of the exercise.

Start

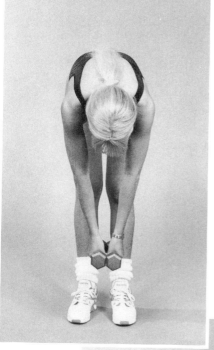

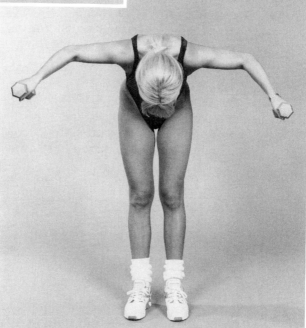

Finish

BICEPS ROUTINE:
SIMULTANEOUS CURL, HAMMER CURL, CONCENTRATION CURL

Do three giant sets of ten repetitions of each of these exercises.

1. Simultaneous Curl

This exercise develops and shapes the entire biceps muscle, and strengthens the forearm.

START: Stand with your feet a natural width apart with a dumbbell in each hand, palms facing away from your body. Place your arms down at your sides, elbows slightly bent, and hold the dumbbells in a horizontal position.

MOVE: Flexing your biceps muscles as you go, and keeping your arms close to the sides of your body, curl your arms upward simultaneously until the dumbbells reach shoulder height and you cannot curl them any further. Keeping the pressure on your biceps muscles, return to the start position and repeat the movement until you have completed your set. Without resting, do your first set of your next biceps exercise, the hammer curl.

TIPS: Don't allow your body to rock as you curl and uncurl the dumbbells. Be sure to perform full repetitions. Go all the way up and all the way down.

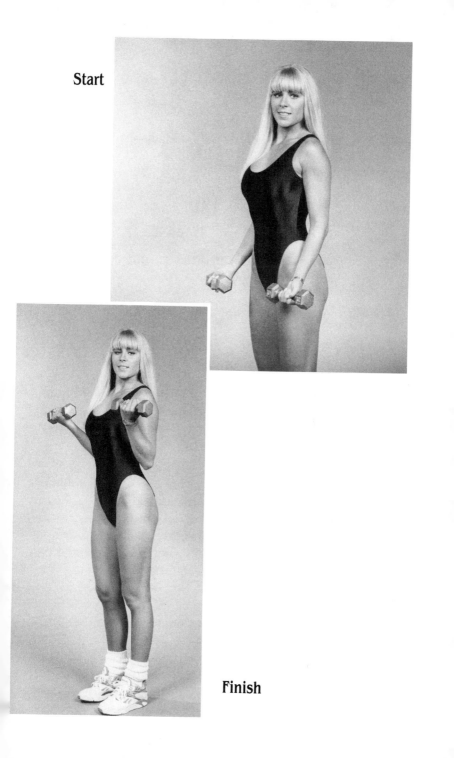

Start

Finish

2. Hammer Curl

This exercise develops, defines, and shapes the entire biceps muscle, and strengthens the forearm.

START: Stand with your feet a natural width apart, with a dumbbell held in each hand, palms facing your body, and with your arms hanging down at either side of your body.

MOVE: With palms facing your body, and the dumbbells in the "hammer" position, curl your right arm up toward your right shoulder. As the dumbbell approaches your right shoulder, begin curling your left arm up toward your left shoulder, and at the same time uncurl your right arm. Continue this alternate curl movement until you have completed your set. Without resting, move to the last biceps exercise, the concentration curl.

TIPS: Keep the pressure on your working biceps muscles at all times, flexing on the up movement and applying dynamic tension on the down movement. Don't rock as you exercise. Keep your body steady. Only your arms should be moving. Don't hold your breath. Breathe naturally.

Start

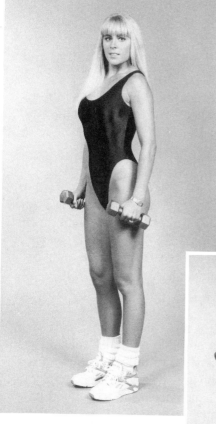

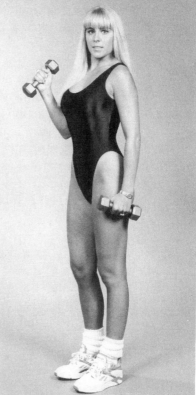

Finish

3. Concentration Curl

This exercise develops, defines, and shapes the entire biceps muscle, especially the peak, and strengthens the forearm.

START: Bend over so that your back is parallel to the floor. Place your right elbow on your right inner knee, holding a dumbbell with palm facing away from your body and arm extended straight down. Support yourself by placing your left hand on your left thigh. (You do not have to hold the dumbbell with your left hand, unless you want to for additional support.)

MOVE: Flexing your biceps muscle as you go, curl your right arm upward until the dumbbell reaches approximate chin height, or until you cannot curl it any further. Applying dynamic tension, return to the start position and repeat the movement until you have completed your set. Perform the set for your other arm. Rest fifteen seconds and do your second and then third giant sets of your biceps routine. Then rest fifteen seconds and begin your triceps routine.

TIPS: Maintain your elbow-on-the-inner-knee position throughout the exercise. Keep your mind on your biceps muscle as you work. You may touch your biceps muscle with your free hand as you exercise, to feel that muscle working. You may also perform this exercise seated in a chair, at the edge of a bed or sofa, or at the edge of an exercise bench.

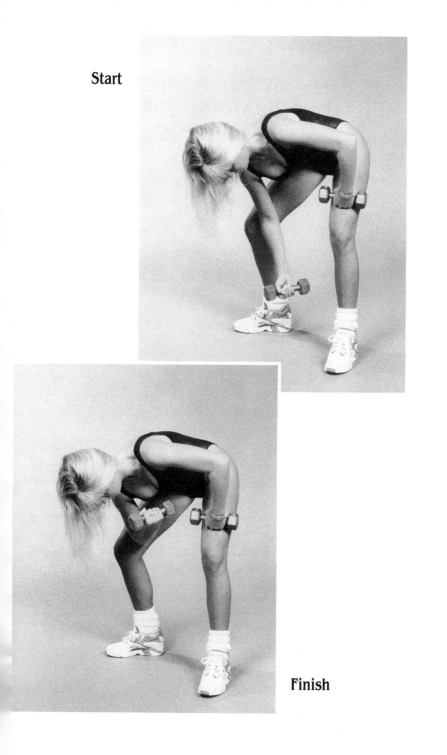

Start

Finish

TRICEPS ROUTINE:
ONE-ARM EXTENSION, KICKBACK,
CROSS-FACE EXTENSION

Do three giant sets of ten repetitions for each exercise.

1. One-Arm Extension

This exercise develops and shapes the entire triceps muscle, especially the inner and middle heads of the muscle.

START: Stand with your feet together, holding a dumbbell in one hand. Raise the dumbbell above your head, holding it straight up, palm facing your body. Extend your arm straight up and pin your biceps muscle close to your ears.

MOVE: Applying tension to your working triceps muscle, lower the dumbbell behind your head, until the dumbbell touches the back of your neck. Flexing your triceps muscle as hard as possible, return to the start position and repeat the movement until you have finished your set. Without resting, begin your next triceps exercise, the kickback.

TIPS: It is crucial that you keep your upper arm nearly pinned to your ears as you lower and raise the dumbbell, otherwise you will take the pressure off your working triceps muscle. You may do this two arms at a time.

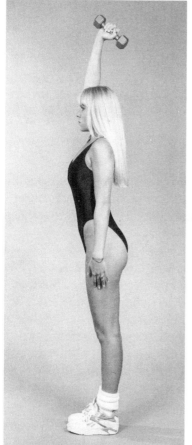

Start

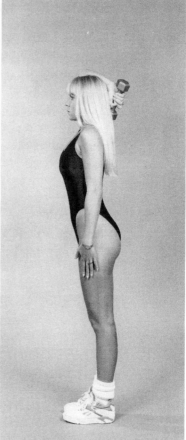

Finish

2. Kickback

This exercise develops, defines, and shapes the entire triceps area, especially the outer head of the muscle.

START: With a dumbbell held in each hand, palms facing your body, bend at the waist and bend your elbows until the dumbbells are held vertically in line with your chest area.

MOVE: Keeping your upper arms close to your body, and flexing your triceps muscle as you go, simultaneously extend your arms behind you until they are fully extended and your elbows are locked. Keeping the tension on your triceps muscle, return to the start and repeat the movement until you have completed your set. Without resting, begin your last triceps exercise, the cross-face extension.

TIPS: Don't hold your breath. Breathe naturally. You may perform this exercise one arm at a time.

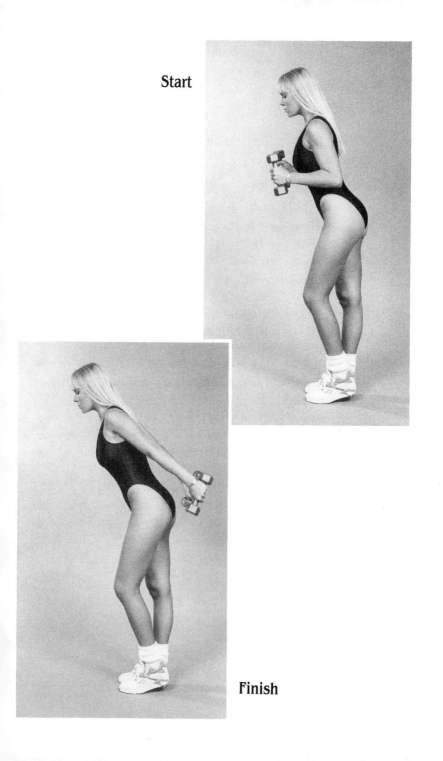

Start

Finish

3. Cross-Face Extension

This exercise develops, defines, and shapes the entire triceps muscle, especially the inner head.

START: Lie on your back on the floor with a dumbbell held in your fully extended right arm, palm facing toward your feet. To avoid hitting yourself in the face, turn your face slightly to the right.

MOVE: Applying dynamic tension as you go, bend your right arm at the elbow, lowering your right arm until the dumbbell touches your left neck-shoulder area. Flexing your right triceps, return to the start position and repeat the movement until you have completed your set. Repeat the set for the other arm. Rest fifteen seconds and then do your second, and then third and final giant sets of your triceps routine. Then rest fifteen seconds and begin your back routine.

TIPS: Don't let your upper arm wander away from the close-to-the-head position as you exercise. Keep your mind on your working triceps muscle throughout the movement.

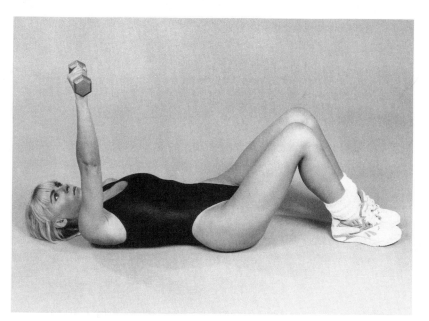

Start

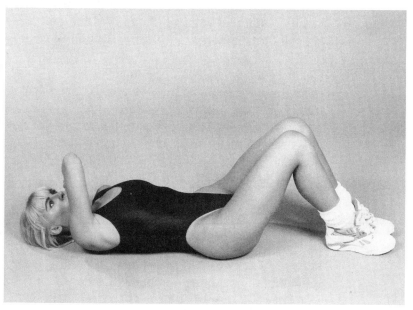

Finish

BACK ROUTINE: REVERSE BENT-DUMBBELL ROW, UPRIGHT ROW, SEATED BACK LATERAL

Do three giant sets of ten repetitions of each exercise.

1. Reverse Bent-Dumbbell Row

This exercise develops, defines, and sculpts the latissimus dorsi (lats) and trapezius muscles.

START: Stand with your feet a natural width apart, holding a dumbbell in each hand, palms facing forward, away from your body. Bend over until your torso is almost parallel with the floor. Hold the dumbbells about six inches out from your body.

MOVE: Flexing your latissimus dorsi muscles as you go, raise the dumbbells as high as possible, keeping them the same six inches away from the sides of your body. Applying dynamic tension to your latissimus dorsi muscles, return to the start position and repeat the movement until you have completed your set. Without resting, move to your next exercise, the upright row.

TIPS: Do not allow yourself to rise from the torso-parallel-to-the-floor position, or you will take the pressure off your working latissimus dorsi muscles. Remember to keep the dumbbells six inches away from the body. It will be easier to do this if you imagine that the dumbbells are a barbell.

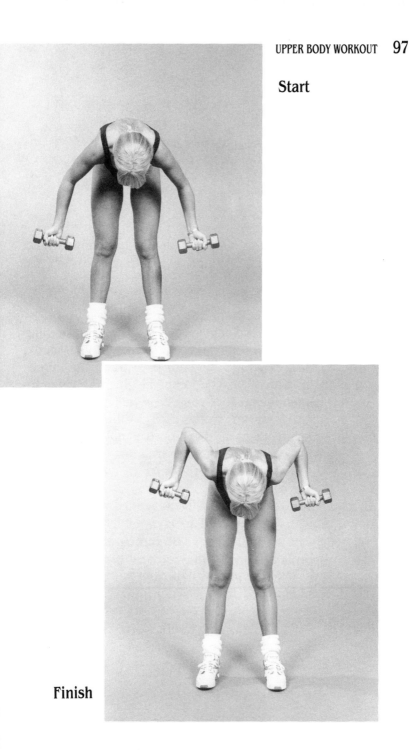

Start

Finish

2. Upright Row

This exercise develops, defines, and shapes the entire trapezius muscle, and helps to develop the anterior (front) deltoid muscle.

START: Stand with your feet together and a dumbbell held with both hands in the center, palms facing your body.

MOVE: Flexing your trapezius and shoulder muscles as you go, extend your elbows outward, and keeping the dumbbell close to the center of your body, and nearly touching your body, raise the dumbbell until it reaches chin height. Applying dynamic tension to your trapezius and shoulder muscles, return to the start position and repeat the movement until you have completed your set. Without resting, move to your last back exercise, the seated back lateral.

TIPS: This exercise is usually performed with a barbell. Once you get used to it, however, a dumbbell becomes quite natural. Be sure to keep the dumbbell close to your body as you exercise, or you will take the pressure off your working trapezius and shoulder muscles.

Start

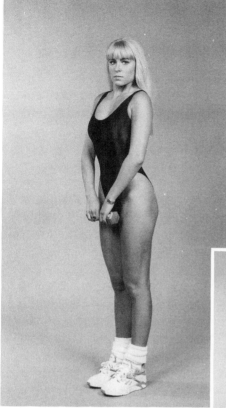

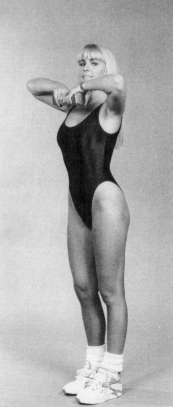

Finish

3. Seated Back Lateral

This exercise develops, defines, and shapes the upper back and trapezius muscles.

START: Sit in a chair, holding a dumbbell in each hand, and lean forward until your upper body is nearly parallel to the floor. Hold the dumbbells, palms facing the back of the chair, behind your lower calves.

MOVE: Flexing your back muscles as you go, and keeping the dumbbells close to your body, raise the dumbbells up and back, rotating the dumbbells as you go along so that when you reach hip level, your palms are facing away from your body. Make believe you are trying to squeeze a pencil in the center of your back, and flex as hard as possible. Applying dynamic tension, return to the start position and repeat the movement until you have completed your set. Rest fifteen seconds and then do your second, then third and final giant sets of your back routine. Congratulations. You have completed your upper body workout.

TIPS: Keep your arms as close to your sides as possible as you move. Let your back stretch out each time you return to the start position.

Start

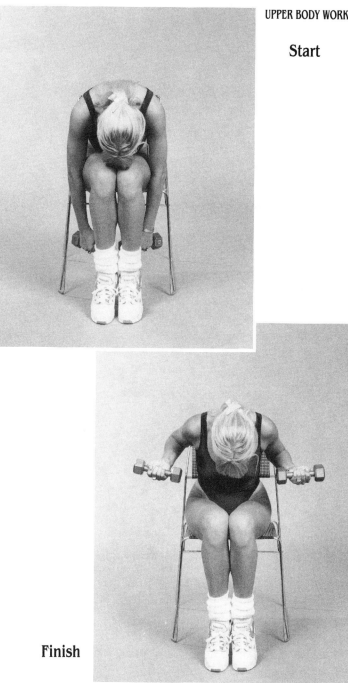

Finish

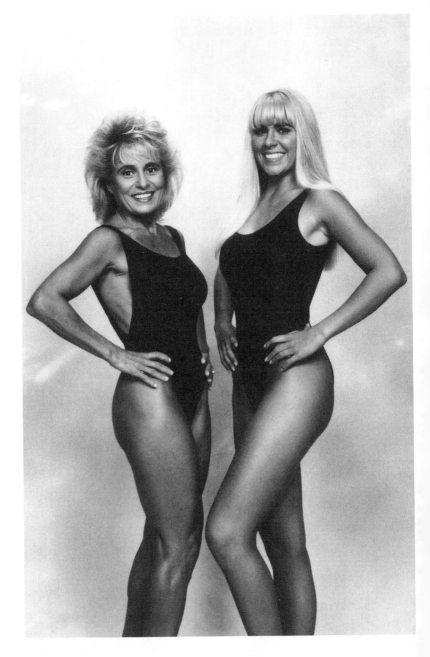

REVIEW OF UPPER BODY EXERCISES

Chest

Incline press
Pec squeeze
Incline flye

Triceps

One-arm extension
Kickback
Cross-face extension

Shoulders

Side lateral
Front lateral
Bent lateral

Back

Reverse bent-dumbbell row
Upright row
Seated back lateral

Biceps

Simultaneous curl
Hammer curl
Concentration curl

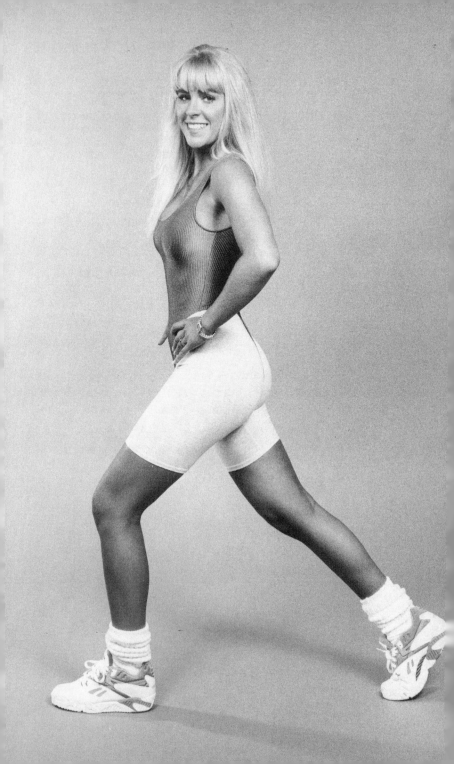

5

LOWER BODY
WORKOUT

Your lower body workout consists of four exercises: thighs, hip-buttocks, abdominals, and calves. But what if you happen to be blessed with beautiful legs? Can you take advantage of this fact and simply skip the thigh routine? No.

This workout is designed to perfect perfection itself. For example, it will sculpt even the most beautiful legs into still more perfect form—putting definition on the front thigh and those indentations on the side that you may have noticed on the legs of models and female athletes.

Even if you have a flat stomach, and your buttocks are not out of control, you should exercise these body parts. The routine will give your stomach definition that will make your waist appear smaller, and will round and lift your buttocks so that they are more appealing than you could have imagined.

What about the calves? Unless you are a runner and have well-developed calves, do the calf routines. Shapely calves make for sexy legs. Years ago, when everyone wore high heels all day, most women had muscular calves. Today, unless a woman is an athlete, she has to work out in order to develop her calves.

You will do three exercises for each lower body part—giant-setting all three exercises of each body part, and at the same time flexing and using dynamic tension so that you get the maximum result from the workout. You will rest fifteen seconds each time you complete a giant set. Follow the exercise instructions and you will be reminded when you can take your fifteen-second rests.

Weights

You will use five-pound dumbbells for all exercises, except for the abdominal exercises, where weights are optional, and the buttocks exercises, where weights are not required. If you find that five-pound dumbbells are not heavy enough, you may advance to eight- or ten-pound dumbbells, but you don't have to do that if you instead choose to compensate by flexing harder and using more dynamic tension, thus making the exercises more challenging.

Note that you will be doing a different number of repetitions for each exercise group, so pay attention to the repetition instructions as each new body part is introduced.

THIGH ROUTINE:
SQUAT, LUNGE, LEG EXTENSION

Do three giant sets of twelve to fifteen repetitions for each of these exercises.

1. Squat

This exercise develops, shapes, and defines the front thigh (quadriceps) muscle, and helps to lift the buttocks (gluteus maximus).

START: With a dumbbell held in each hand, stand with your feet in a natural position. Hold your arms down at your sides, with the dumbbells held palms facing your body. Keep your back straight.

MOVE: Rising slightly up on your toes if necessary, and applying dynamic tension to your front thigh muscles, descend to a squatting position. Flexing your front thigh muscles, return to the start and repeat the movement until you have completed your set. Without resting, proceed to your next thigh exercise, the lunge.

TIPS: If you want to place a greater emphasis on the inner thigh, point your toes outward as far as possible and otherwise perform the exercise as described above. Be careful not to lean forward as you squat. (You may place a two by four piece of wood under your heels if you feel it helps with your balance.)

If you cannot do this exercise because of knee problems, double up on your leg extensions.

Start

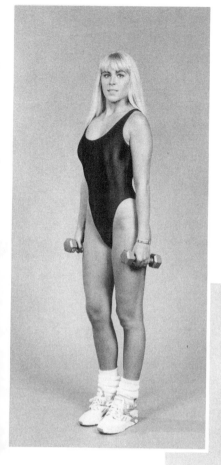

Finish

2. Lunge

This exercise develops, shapes, and defines the front thigh (quadriceps) muscle, and helps to lift and tighten the hips and gluteus maximus (buttocks).

START: Stand with your feet a natural width apart and your back straight, with a dumbbell held in each hand, palms facing your body, and with your arms straight down at your sides.

MOVE: Lunge forward with your right leg, about two and a half feet, or until you cannot lunge any further, bending your left knee as you go. Flexing your left front thigh muscle, return to the start position, and repeat the movement for your other leg. Continue this alternate lunging movement until you have completed a full set for each leg. Without resting, proceed to your final leg exercise, the leg extension.

TIPS: Don't look down at your legs, or you will lose your balance. Don't bounce off the nonlunging leg. Make your movements deliberate. Don't worry if you wobble and lose balance for the first few weeks. This is natural. In time, you will have no problem. For a greater emphasis on the inner thigh, point the toes of your lunging leg as far outward as possible.

   If you can't do this exercise because of knee problems, double or triple up on the next exercise, the leg extension.

Start

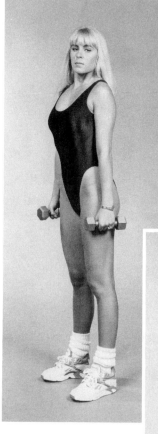

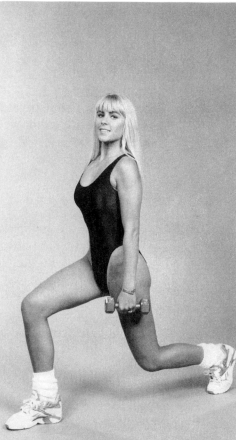

Finish

3. Leg Extension

This exercise develops, shapes, and defines the front thigh (quadriceps) muscle.

START: Sit in a chair or on a stable flat surface with a dumbbell held between your feet. Hold on to the chair on either side of you, and lean back about six inches, arching your back slightly.

MOVE: Flex your front thigh (quadriceps) muscle and extend your legs straight out in front of you until they are parallel to the floor or higher. Apply dynamic tension as you return to the start position, keeping continual pressure on your front thigh muscle. Repeat the movement until you have finished your set. Rest fifteen seconds and then do your second and then third giant sets of this routine. Then rest fifteen seconds and begin your hip-buttocks routine.

TIPS: If you try to do this exercise sitting on the edge of a bed, you will find it is difficult to get the full tension in your working leg, because the bed will not be stable. But if you have no other choice, a bed will do. Once you get used to compensating for the instability of the bed, you will be able to control your flexing quite well.

Start

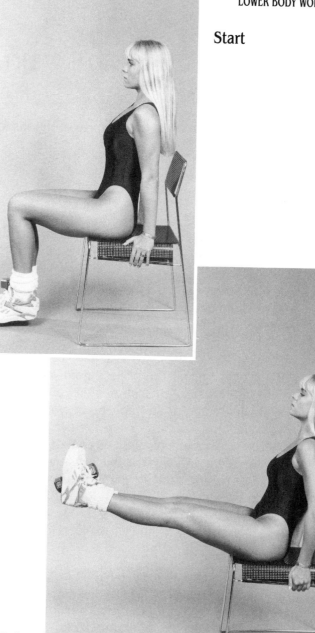

Finish

HIP-BUTTOCKS ROUTINE: FEATHER KICK-UP, ONE-LEGGED BUTT LIFT, SCISSORS

Do three giant sets of fifteen to twenty-five repetitions for each of these exercises.

1. Feather Kick-up

This exercise lifts, tightens, and tones the entire hip-buttocks area, and helps to tighten the back thigh.

START: Get on the floor in an all-fours position. Raise your right leg up and bend at the knee so that your leg takes the shape of an L.

MOVE: Pointing your toes toward the ceiling, and applying the maximum of flexing power on your right hip-buttocks area, straighten your right leg by raising your leg and unbending your knee at the same time. Continue this movement until your knee is no longer bent, and you cannot raise your leg any higher. Using dynamic tension, return to the start position and repeat the movement until you have completed your set. Repeat the set for the other leg. Without resting, move on to your next hip-buttocks exercise, the one-legged butt lift.

TIPS: You must return to the L position each time you unbend your leg. Don't be discouraged if this exercise seems awkward and hard to learn at first. It is the most effective hip-buttocks exercise. Soon you will love it.

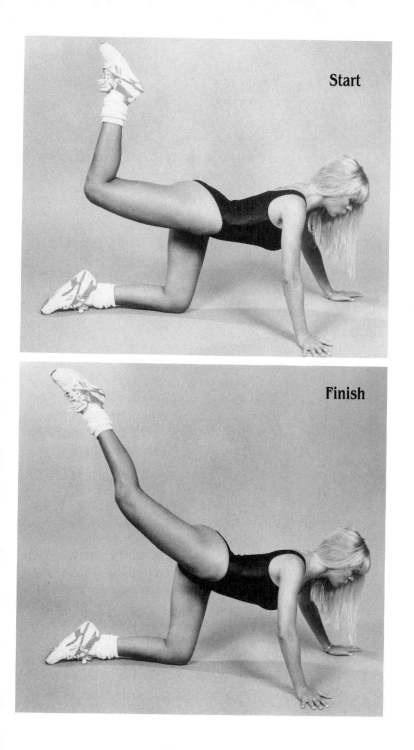

Start

Finish

2. One-Legged Butt Lift

This exercise lifts, tightens, and tones the entire hip-buttocks area and helps to tighten the back thigh (biceps femoris, or hamstring) muscle.

START: Facing a holding object, such as a chair, desk, or bed, kneel with your right leg slightly bent at the knee. Extend your arms and grasp the holding object with both hands on either side.

MOVE: Flexing your right hip-buttocks area as hard as possible, point your right toes behind you and extend your leg straight out behind you. Continuing to keep the pressure on your right hip-buttocks area, return to the start position and repeat the movement until you have completed your set. Repeat the exercise for your other leg. Without resting, move on to your final hip-buttocks exercise, the scissors.

TIPS: Don't bend your back as your work. Keep it as straight as possible. It's okay to lean slightly to the side opposite your working leg. Remember to squeeze your entire hip-buttocks area as you work. It's the pressure you apply that tightens your hip-buttocks, as well as the movement. If it is more convenient, you may do this movement standing up.

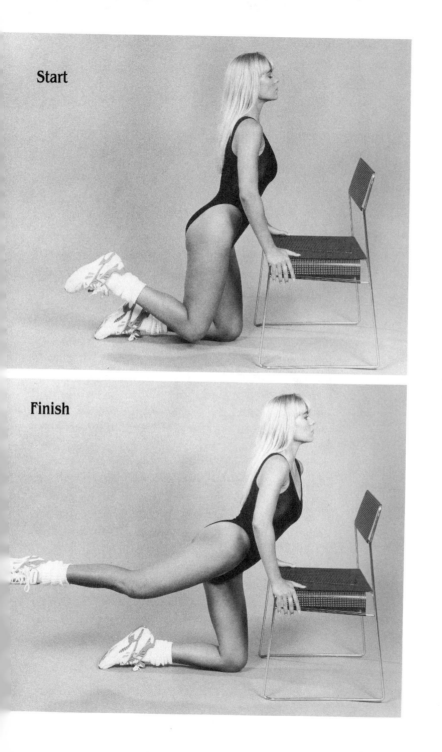

Start

Finish

3. Scissors

This exercise lifts, tightens, and tones the entire hip-buttocks area and helps to tighten and define the front and back thigh muscles.

START: Lay back on a chair or a stable area (you can do this seated on your desk top) with your palms facing down, under each buttock. Extend your legs straight out in front of you until your knees are locked. Point your toes forward.

MOVE: Squeezing your hip-buttocks area as hard as possible, scissor your legs apart until you cannot go any further. (You should be able to feel the complete flexing of your buttocks with your hands.) Keeping the pressure on your entire buttocks area, return to the start, touching your heels together, but not crossing your legs over each other. Continue this scissorslike movement until you have completed your set. Rest fifteen seconds and then do your second and then third giant sets of your hip-buttocks routine. Then rest fifteen seconds and move on to your abdominal routine.

TIPS: This is a very simple, yet very effective exercise. It's a good idea to take advantage of its ease and do twenty-five repetitions. Remember to use continual tension as you work.

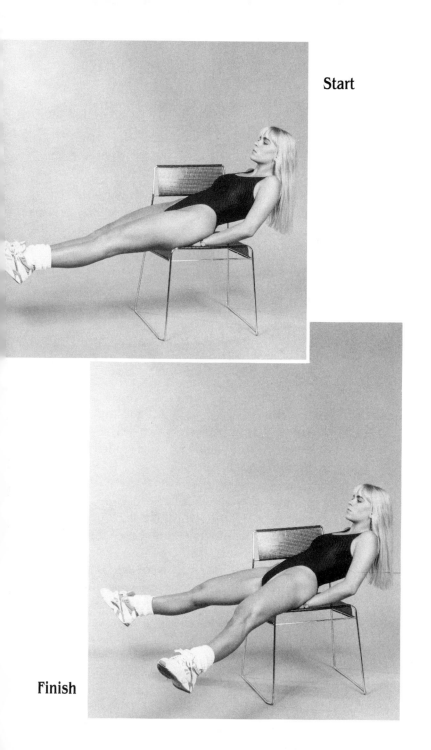

Start

Finish

ABDOMINAL ROUTINE: BENT-KNEE SIT-UP (OR CRUNCH), KNEE-IN (OR REVERSE CRUNCH), OBLIQUE CRUNCH

You will do three giant sets of fifteen to twenty-five repetitions for each of these exercises. For those of you who have back problems, note the alternate suggestions in the tips sections, or the fully explained alternate exercises.

1. Bent-Knee Sit-up

This exercise defines, flattens, and strengthens the upper abdominal area, and will eventually result in washboard-flat abdominals.

START: Lie on the floor, flat on your back, and bend your knees so that the soles of your feet are flat on the floor. Place your hands on your stomach, or place them behind your head.

MOVE: Flexing your upper abdominal muscles as hard as possible, raise yourself off the floor until you are sitting up. (The movement is one of curling rather than jerking.) Keeping the pressure on your upper abdominal muscles, return to the start position, and without bouncing off the floor repeat the movement until you have completed your set. Without resting, proceed to your next abdominal exercise, the knee-in.

TIPS: It may take awhile to be able to do a full fifteen repetitions. Start with as many as you can com-

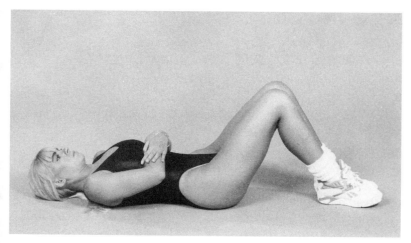

Start

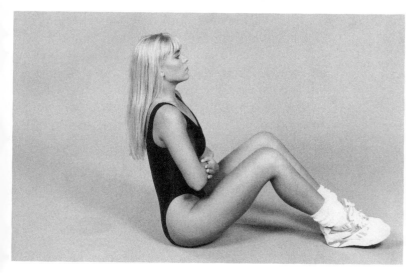

Finish

fortably do and add one repetition to each workout until you have come up to the full fifteen. If you
cannot perform this exercise, you may replace it
with the crunch. See the next page for this exercise.

Alternative for Bent-Knee Sit-up: Crunch

This exercise tightens and tones the entire upper abdominal area. It also helps to strengthen the lower back.

START: Lie flat on your back on the floor, and bend your knees until the soles of your feet are flat on the ground. Place your hands behind your head or folded and placed on your stomach.

MOVE: Raise your shoulders until they are completely off the ground, all the time flexing your upper abdominal muscles as hard as possible. Without letting up on the tension, return to the start position and repeat the movement until you have finished your set. Without pausing, move to your next abdominal exercise, the knee-in (or the reverse crunch).

TIPS: Do not rise to a sitting position. This is a crunch, not a sit-up. Rise only to shoulders-off-the-ground level.

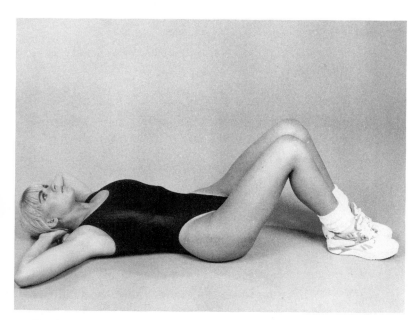

Start

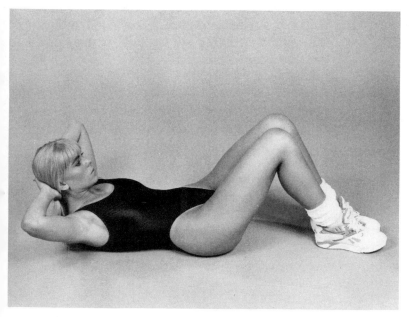

Finish

2. Knee-in

This exercise defines, flattens, and strengthens the entire lower abdominal area, and helps to strengthen the lower back.

START: Lie on the floor, flat on your back, and extend your legs and knees, with ankles crossed, straight out in front of you.

MOVE: Flexing your lower abdominal muscles as hard as possible, pull your knees toward your chest until you cannot go any further. Keeping the pressure on your lower abdominal muscles, return to the start position and repeat the movement until you have completed your set. Without resting, move to your last abdominal exercise, the oblique crunch.

TIPS: Keep your knees and ankles together as you work. This will force greater pressure to be exerted on the lower abdominal area, and you will see greater results. Keep your mind on your lower abdominal area as you exercise. Don't hold your breath. Breathe naturally. If you cannot do this exercise, do the alternative, the reverse crunch.

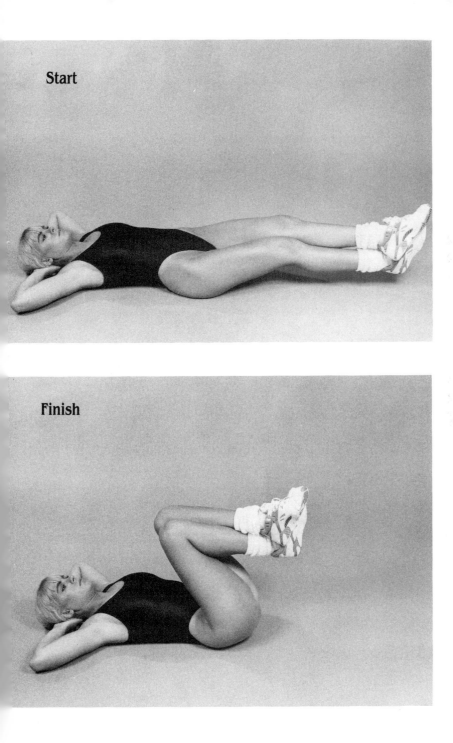

Start

Finish

Alternative for Knee-in: Reverse Crunch

This exercise defines, tightens, and strengthens the lower abdominal area, and also strengthens the lower back muscles.

START: Lie on the floor flat on your back with your knees completely bent (to approximately a 90 degree angle). You may place your hands at your sides, behind your head, or under your buttocks for support. Cross your legs at the ankles.

MOVE: Flexing your lower abdominal muscles as hard as possible, raise your lower abdominal area by lifting your pelvic area and bringing your knees toward your face. Without pausing, and keeping the pressure on your lower abdominal muscles, return to the start position and repeat the movement until you have completed your set. Without resting, move to your final abdominal exercise, the oblique crunch.

TIPS: Don't merely bounce off the floor as you raise your lower abdominals. Make your movements deliberate and controlled. Keep your mind on your lower abdominal muscles throughout the exercise. Don't hold your breath. Breathe naturally.

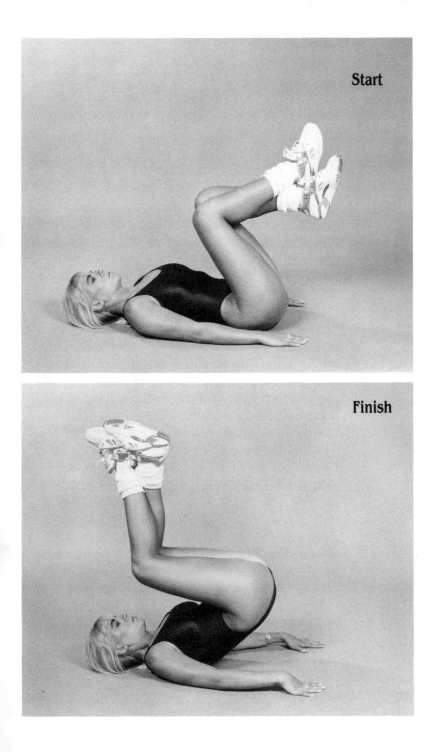

Start

Finish

3. Oblique Crunch

This exercise defines, flattens, and strengthens the side abdominal (oblique) muscles (love handles will soon go), as well as the upper and lower abdominal muscles.

START: Lie on the floor flat on your back and bend your knees. Place your feet together and let your legs fall to one side until you knees are touching the floor. Place your hands behind your head.

MOVE: Keeping your back as parallel to the ceiling as possible, raise your shoulders (not your back) off the floor until you are in the crunch position. Be sure to move up in a straight line and to lift from the chest and not the neck. Keeping the pressure on your working oblique muscle, repeat the movement until you have completed your set. Repeat the set for the other side of your body. Rest fifteen seconds and then do your second and then third giant sets for this routine. Then rest fifteen seconds and move to your calf routine.

TIPS: Keep your shoulders lined up as parallel to the floor as possible as you move. Your chest should be facing straight to the ceiling throughout the movement. Place your fingertips on your working oblique muscles and feel the flex of your oblique muscles.

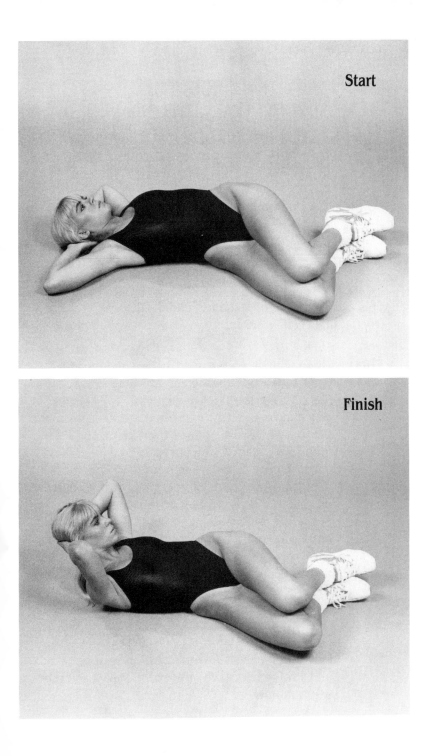

Start

Finish

CALF ROUTINE:
SEATED STRAIGHT-TOE RAISE,
SEATED ANGLED-OUT TOE RAISE,
SEATED ANGLED-IN TOE RAISE

Do three sets of ten repetitions for each exercise.

1. Seated Straight-Toe Raise

This exercise develops, shapes, and defines the entire gastrocnemius (calf) muscle.

START: Sit on a chair, with a dumbbell on your knees and your toes on a dictionary or other thick book, the spine of the book facing you. Let your heels descend as low to the ground as possible. Hold the dumbbell with your favored hand, and let the other hand dangle at your side.

MOVE: Keeping your toes pointed straight ahead, raise up on your toes as high as possible. When you reach the high point, flex your calf muscles as hard as possible and, continuing to exert pressure, return to the start position, letting your calf muscles stretch out to the fullest extent. Repeat the movement until you have completed your set. Without resting, proceed to your next calf exercise, the seated angled-out toe raise.

TIPS: Don't bounce up or drop down on your toes. Flex and stretch with each movement. Make each repetition count.

Start

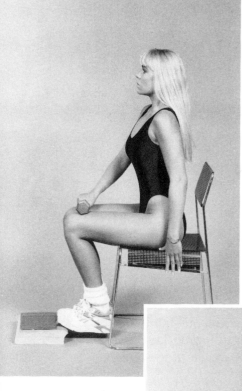

Finish

2. Seated Angled-Out Toe Raise

This exercise develops, shapes, and defines the entire gastrocnemius muscle, especially the inner calf area.

START: Place your toes on a dictionary or thick book, with your toes angled out to the side (away from your body) as far as possible. Place a dumbbell on your lap. Lower your heels to the floor as far as possible.

MOVE AND TIPS: Follow the instructions for the seated straight-toe raise on the previous page. After completing this exercise, without resting, do your last calf exercise, the seated angled-in toe raise.

3. Seated Angled-In Toe Raise

This exercise develops, defines, and shapes the entire calf (gastrocnemius) muscle, especially the outer calf area.

START: Place your toes on a dictionary or thick book, with your heels as low to the ground as possible. Point your toes inward as far as possible and keep them that way throughout the movement. Place a dumbbell on your lap.

MOVE AND TIPS: Perform this exercise in the same manner as the seated straight-toe raise (see page 130), only keep your toes pointed inward throughout the movement. After you have completed this exercise, rest fifteen seconds and then do a second and then third giant set for this routine. Congratulations, you have completed your lower body workout.

REVIEW OF LOWER BODY EXERCISES

Thighs

Squat
Lunge
Leg extension

Hip-Buttocks

Feather kick-up
One-legged butt lift
Scissors

Abdominals

Bent-knee sit-up (or crunch)
Knee-in (or reverse crunch)
Oblique crunch

Calves

Seated straight-toe raise
Seated angled-out toe raise
Seated angled-in toe raise

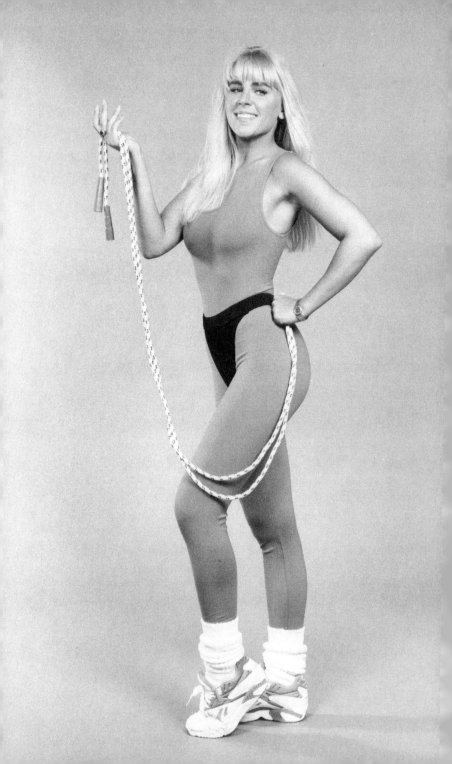

6

AEROBICS

Most people enjoy aerobics. You don't really have to concentrate when you perform an aerobic activity. You can just let your mind wander. After a while, it doesn't even seem like work, and you're burning fat all along. In addition, there is a natural high that comes with such exercise. (Also, with aerobics, once you get used to the activity, you don't have to think or concentrate at all as you exercise. It's almost as if you turn on a switch and you go on automatic.)

Aerobic exercises are excellent for balancing out your workout, because when you run, bike, swim, or jump rope, for example, you give your heart and lungs a real workout. True, you do get an aerobic workout with the weight-training program put forth in this book, but the fact is, if you take advantage of the fifteen-second rests, there is a slight interruption in the aerobic flow. So unless you hate aerobics, or unless you just love the weight program so much that you want to do nothing but the weights, it's a good idea to balance out your workout with straight aerobics.

WHAT MAKES AN ACTIVITY AEROBIC?

In order to be considered aerobic, an exercise must involve the movement of the large muscles of the body in a continual, rhythmic manner for twenty minutes or more, and it must keep the pulse rate up to between 60 percent and 85 percent of capacity.

Whether an exercise is aerobic or anaerobic is based upon the way the body uses oxygen during that activity. An aerobic exercise is supported by the body's ongoing supply of oxygen. An anaerobic activity, on the other hand, cannot be supported by the body's natural supply of oxygen because such an activity is too strenuous. One must periodically stop for air or oxygen.

If you don't take too many rests, the College Dorm Workout keeps your heart rate between 60 percent and 70 percent of capacity, the ideal fat-burning range. But some people wonder: since the College Dorm Workout is a weight-training routine, how can it be considered an aerobic activity? Isn't it true that weight training has always been considered anaerobic?

Weight training is an anaerobic activity when heavy weights are used, because lifting heavy weights is so strenuous that one must rest for relatively long periods of time after each set of lifting. With the College Dorm Workout, you rest little or not at all, so your exercise is aerobic.

STRAIGHT AEROBIC CHOICES

As mentioned above, however, since periodic rests are allowed, if you like straight aerobics, it is a good idea to use Plan A and to include three sessions of straight aerobics in your weekly routine. How will you decide which aerobic activity to choose? You'll have to combine three factors: enjoyment, convenience, and fat burning.

For your information, here is a chart that tells you how much fat is burned during a twenty-minute session of various aerobic activities.

Chances are, even if you like certain activities better than others, and even if certain activities burn more fat than others, you will have to make your decision based upon convenience. The following aerobic choices are discussed in order of their probable convenience.

Running, Race Walking, Jogging, Walking at a Fast Pace

When it comes to walking, race walking, or jogging as opposed to running, the same amount of fat can be burned—only you'll have to do it longer, depending upon which activity you choose. Look at the chart. Notice that the chart points out that you will burn 110 calories after twenty minutes of walking, but 220 calories after running a nine-minute mile. You will have to walk double the time you would have had to run to get the same amount of fat burning.

Running, race walking, jogging, and walking at a fast pace are ideal aerobic activities for their convenience and for the opportunity they give you to enjoy the outdoors.

AEROBIC EXERCISE CHART

Aerobic Activity	Calories Burned per 20 Minutes
The College Dorm Workout	240
Stair machine	260
Running 8-minute mile	230
Running 9-minute mile	220
Cross-country skiing	220
Swimming	210
Stair stepping	200
Rope jumping	200
Low-impact aerobics (aerobic dance)	200
Nordic Track machine	165
Race walking	160
Rowing machine	150
Jogging at easy pace	145
Bicycle riding	140
Moderate dance—freestyle	120
Walking fast pace	110

Running is the most challenging of these activities, but race walking is a close second. Serious race walkers use up almost as much energy as runners, because not only do they move at a rapid pace, but they constantly flex their muscles as they go. Jogging falls in between walking and running in energy expenditure. It's actually running at a very easy pace. Walking fast is the most relaxing of the above. The best part about walking is you can kill two birds with one stone. You can walk to a destination—say a friend's dorm at the other side of the campus, a twenty-minute walk each way—and you've accomplished your aerobic workout for the day. (Remember, you have to double the time if you're walking. Yes. You can break it up into twenty minutes each way if you choose walking.)

Rope Jumping

You can jump rope in the privacy of your own room while watching television or listening to music, and all you need is an inexpensive jump rope. (Even a child's rope will do.) If you're a private person, and perhaps don't relish the idea of having people see you huffing and puffing as you run around the campus or the track, rope jumping can be a godsend.

Rope jumping not only gets your heart and lungs in shape and helps to burn fat, but it gives your shoulders, arms, back, and legs quite a workout.

Stationary Bike and Stair-Stepper

If you have the room, you can get an inexpensive stationary bicycle or stair-stepper, keep it in your room, and work out while you study, read, watch television, or some such thing.

If you choose one of these machines, don't set the tension so high that you are straining after two minutes. Keep the tension at the lowest level so that you can enjoy your workout. There's no need to get your heart up to the 85 percent range. In fact, it has been determined by the medical profession that the ideal fat-burning range is between 60 percent and 70 percent of the maximum. You don't have to scientifically monitor yourself to know if you have reached this level. You are at it when you can speak with someone, but not carry on an animated, relaxed conversation. Also, you are at this level when you break a sweat after about five to seven minutes of working out.

These machines challenge the lower body—the thighs, hips, and buttocks. The bike challenges the thighs more than the hip-buttocks area, and the stair machine challenges the hip-buttocks area more than the thighs.

If you choose either one of these machines, you should be aware that they cannot reshape your thighs, hips, or buttocks; they can only help to burn fat and reduce the size of these areas. For perfect shaping, you will have to do the lower body workout.

Swimming

Most colleges have a pool, so if you like the water, why not swim? Nearly every muscle in your body is involved when you swim, but the muscles most challenged are the chest, shoulder, back, and abdominal muscles. Swimming is also great if you've sustained an injury and cannot do anything else, because with swimming, there is almost no stress on the muscles, bones, and joints.

If you really want to burn maximum fat when you swim, don't do the easier strokes such as the backstroke or the sidestroke. Instead, do the crawl or the butterfly.

Rowing Machine, Nordic Track Machine, Treadmill

Chances are, your college has a gym with some aerobic equipment. If you feel like getting away from it all and going to the college gym, you can take advantage of the rowing machines, the Nordic Track machine, or the treadmill.

The rowing machine helps to build upper body strength and endurance. It challenges mainly the chest, shoulders, back, biceps, and even triceps. Some lower body work is involved (your legs and buttocks are moving). However, as mentioned before, you will still have to work with weights to develop and shape your upper body muscles into perfect form.

The Nordic Track machine combines both upper and lower body work, and helps to build strength and endurance for the entire body. It is a very challenging workout. That's why you rarely see a line forming at this machine!

The treadmill has nearly the same effect as running, but with some advantages and some disadvantages. With the treadmill, you can set an even pace and make sure that you keep it because your clocked-in speed will force you to do so. Also, you can raise or lower your pace at will, but all the time you will know exactly how much fat you are burning.

The disadvantage of the treadmill as opposed to running is that running outside makes your body work a little harder. You tend to raise your legs higher and to leap into the run just a bit more. You can of course compensate for this disadvantage by setting the treadmill at a very high speed, but that's no fun! Also, the treadmill can be considered to be boring as compared to running, because outdoors, at least you can enjoy the changing scenery.

Aerobic Dance and Step Aerobics

If your college offers aerobic dance or a step aerobic class, and if your schedule allows you to go, and you like these activities, perfect! They are excellent aerobic choices. Not only do you burn fat and challenge your muscles, but you get to have some fun with other people. In addition, because you're not doing it alone, the time goes faster, and before you know it, it's over.

Aerobic dance challenges nearly all the muscles in the body, and helps to build muscular endurance. Step aerobics strengthens the thighs and hip-buttocks area, but does little for the upper body.

The biggest problem with step aerobics is that people foolishly believe this activity will shape their thighs and buttocks into perfect form, when all it can do is help burn overall body fat and reduce the overall size of these areas.

Cross-Country Skiing

If you are a college student, you will certainly not be able to use cross-country skiing as a regular aerobic activity, but if you happen to get away for a weekend, and you cross-country ski, you can count it as one aerobic workout because it keeps your heart rate well within the ideal fat-burning range for a lot more than twenty minutes.

The steady, rhythmic pace of this activity, which utilizes all major muscles (arms, shoulders, chest, back, stomach, hips, buttocks, and legs are all moving), gives it its aerobic component.

Fast Social Dancing

Since this is the most convenient aerobic exercise of all, you may be wondering why it wasn't listed first. The fact is, in order for dancing to be considered an aerobic activity, it has to be done at a brisk pace and for twenty minutes without stopping (except for a few seconds). If you are the type who dances for five minutes and then stands around for two hours, forget about counting this as your aerobic activity. If, however, you get up on the floor and stay there for hours, this is a perfect aerobic exercise for you. Any fast-moving dancing counts for aerobics.

Dancing challenges most of the muscles of the body, and is so much fun that you don't think of it as exercise at all. Chances are you will not go dancing more than once or twice a week, but when you do, you can count dancing as an aerobic session.

YOU CAN DO ANY COMBINATION OF AEROBICS!

If you have chosen Plan A or C and want to do three sessions of aerobics weekly, you can do any combination of the above. If you like to do the same thing each time, pick your favorite and do it. If you hate a steady routine, you can continually switch from one activity to another. The choice is yours.

CAN YOU TRIPLE-UP ON AN AEROBIC SESSION?

What if you dance or do an aerobic activity for more than twenty minutes—can you count it for more than one session? No. For example, if you dance for an hour, you cannot count it as three twenty-minute aerobic sessions. Be happy that you burned a great deal of calories in that hour, but realize that you must still do aerobics on two additional days.

CAN YOU COUNT YOUR SPORT AS AN AEROBIC ACTIVITY?

In order for your sport to count as an aerobic activity, it would have to be very aerobic in nature. The most aerobic sports are lacrosse, ice or field hockey, soccer, rowing, canoeing, roller skating, roller blading, ice skating, and basketball. Next in line are softball, handball, and racquetball. Tennis and volleyball do burn some fat, but because you are regularly stopping, they really can't be counted as aerobic activities.

The rule of thumb is if your sport keeps you continually on the move, you can count it as an aerobic activity. Use the guideline above and your own judgment as to whether or not your sport counts for an aerobic session.

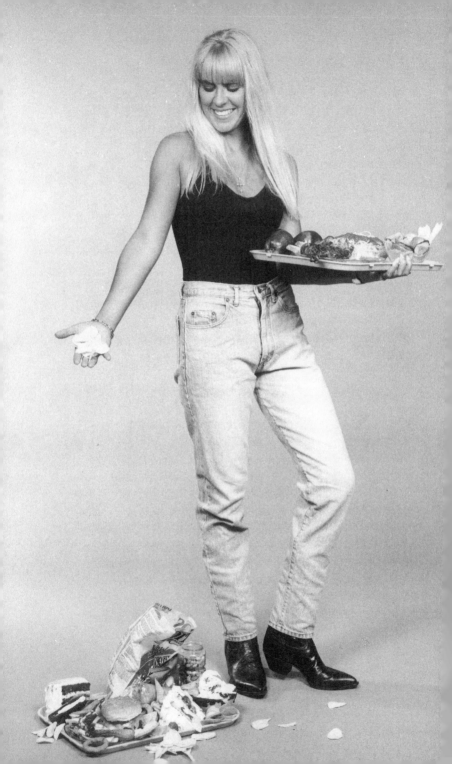

7

CAMPUS EATING WITHOUT GETTING FAT—OR STARVING TO DEATH!

The workout is half the battle—what you eat is the other half. But just as surprisingly simple as it is to get in shape by working out the right way, it's simple to lose weight (fat) and keep it off by eating the right way—and without starving to death.

In the following paragraphs we'll review the basic facts about food so that you will know once and for all how much of which foods you can eat in order to be healthy, strong, and most of all, lean and gorgeous! No longer will you feel guilty about everything you put in your mouth, because finally you'll realize that certain foods simply cannot make you fat.

CALORIES, AND HOW WE GET FAT

Calories are fuel, the units of chemical energy released to our bodies through the food we eat. Just the way a car would refuse to start without gas, or would sputter and stop if it ran out of gas, the body would stop functioning if we didn't supply it with calories.

But that's where the car and human analogy end. A car has no system for storing extra gas. If you try to overfill the gas tank, the excess gas would neither go into the tank, nor would it be stored in another place. It would spill to the ground. On the other hand, if you try to overfill your body with food (calories) your body *will* take them in because it does have a system for storing them as fuel for future use. It stores them in the form of fat. The body's main storage tanks for fat, especially on women, are the hips, the buttocks, the thighs, and the stomach. When these tanks are full, the body begins to store fat all over— on the arms, the back, the face, and eventually even in the most unlikely places, such as the neck, the hands, or the feet.

The body does this as part of its natural survival system—storing the fat so that in case you deprive it of food in the future it will be able to stay alive by using that reserve. But (since it is very unlikely that there will be a famine) in America, most of us don't need or want a hefty fat reserve all over our bodies. In fact, we'd be happy if we had no fat reserve at all.

HOW TO LOSE WEIGHT AND KEEP IT OFF

But since most of us do have a fat reserve, how can we get rid it? We must use up the stored fat by creating a calorie deficit, thus forcing the body to go into its fat reserve, but we must do this in a slow, steady fashion—not by going on a starvation diet; otherwise, when we are off guard, the body's survival system will take over and sabotage our plans, and force us to eat without control until it has regained all of the lost fat—with some additional fat in the bargain! This is a very crucial point and must be remembered at all times. When it comes to losing weight, there are no shortcuts. As the saying goes, you can't fool mother nature.

In order to lose one pound of fat, you must create a calorie deficit of 3,500 calories. You can do this by eating less food than your body would need on a given day even if you didn't exercise; and then, on top of that, by exercising in order to further increase the calorie deficit; and finally, by putting permanent muscle on your body so that more calories will automatically be burned twenty-four hours a day.

Everyone burns calories twenty-four hours a day, even while sleeping, but muscular people burn more calories, even during sleep, than do nonmuscular people. For example, the average nonmuscular person burns about about sixty calories an hour while sleeping, while the average muscular person burns about eighty calories an hour while sleeping.

SIX RULES FOR LOSING WEIGHT AND KEEPING IT OFF

In order to lose weight, and keep it off, you will not only have to create a calorie deficit, but you will have to observe some simple rules of nutritious eating and living that will encourage your body to cooperate with you and to give up its excess fat. Rules 1 through 5 will be discussed here. We've already discussed No. 6.

1. Keep your fat intake low—between twenty and thirty grams per day.
2. Eat two to three portions of low-fat protein per day.
3. Eat three to five portions of limited complex carbohydrates a day, and two to four fruits a day.
4. To stave off hunger, choose filling foods that are high in caloric density, such as baked potatoes, other vegetables, oatmeal, pasta, and rice.
5. Never go more than four to five hours without eating or your metabolism will slow down and you will hinder your weight loss. Eat unlimited complex carbohydrates (vegetables, see list on page 166) whenever you are hungry.
6. Do the College Dorm Workout to burn calories and add permanent muscularity that will speed up your metabolism so that you can eat more without getting fat.

By following these rules, you will be able to create a daily calorie deficit that will force your body to use up (burn off) its stored fat so that you will get to your goal weight, and when you get there will allow you to stay there, because you have not punished and threatened it with starvation diets. Now let's analyze the rules so that they become second nature.

Rule No. 1: Keep Your Fat Intake Low: Between Twenty and Thirty Grams

The fact is, some calories are fatter than others, and as you might have guessed, fat is the fattest of them all. There are only four calories per gram of carbohydrate and protein, but there are nine calories per gram of fat. Fat, then, is more than twice as fat as protein or carbohydrate. But fat is even fatter than that.

When you consume a fatty food, such as potato chips or fried foods, only 2 percent to 3 percent of the fat in those foods is used up in the digestion process. But when you ingest a low-fat protein or carbohydrate food, such as tuna in water or a plain baked potato, 15 percent to 25 percent of the calories are used up in the digestion process.

Let's look at a specific example. If you consume 100 calories in fat, ninety-seven or ninety-eight of those calories are available to use as energy or stored fat, but if you consume 100 calories in carbohydrates or protein, only 75 to 85 of those calories are available for use as energy or stored fat. So when you eat a greasy hamburger or a bag of corn chips, you might as well tack those foods right on to your hips, buttocks, stomach, and thighs, because that's exactly where they go—and quite directly.

FAT IS NOT ALL BAD!

Fat, of course, isn't all bad. We do need a certain amount of it in our diet because our cell membranes and sex hormones are made of fat, and our internal organs are protected by a cushion of surrounding fat. Fat also helps the body to utilize certain minerals and vitamins.

So don't get any bright ideas about completely eliminating fat from your diet. You probably couldn't do that anyway even if you wanted to, because there is at least a trace of fat in most foods. Even an apple has a gram of fat.

RED ALERT: NO-NOS UNTIL YOU REACH YOUR GOAL

The following foods are composed of more than 50 percent fat, and are completely off limits until you reach your weight goal, when you can have them once a week if you desire. Avoid all of these foods, or foods that contain them.

If you are about to consume a food that is not on this list, and you are in doubt as to whether a food is too high in fat, check the food label, or refer to a fat-gram counter such as the one listed on pages 153–155. Any food that is more than 30 percent fat is too high in fat for your purposes, but you don't have to think in terms of percentages since you will be counting fat grams. You cannot exceed thirty grams of fat on any given day and you should try to keep it to twenty. That is all you really need to know.

FAT BANDITS

Butter	Sour cream	Lamb	Fried foods
Margarine	Cream cheese	Veal	Poultry skin
Lard	Cheese	Nuts	Chocolate
Oil	Bacon	Olives	Donuts
Mayonnaise	Beef	Avocados	Ice cream
Chips (potato, corn, etc.)			

FAT FOOD VILLAINS THAT SABOTAGE THE COLLEGE STUDENT'S DIET

There are certain seemingly innocent munchies that college students like to eat. Many of them are not very filling, so you can eat quite a bit of them before you realize you have done any damage. When you look at the following list, you'll see how easy it would be to consume more than five times your ideal fat allowance (20 times 5, or 100 grams of fat).

Favorite Fatty Food Munchie	**Fat Grams**
4 ounces potato chips	45
4 ounces tortilla chips	30
4 ounces Fritos corn chips	36
4 ounces cheese puff balls	40
4 ounces cheese crackers	40
4 ounces peanuts	35
10 chocolate sandwich cookies	34
McDonald's apple pie	14
Chocolate candy bar	15
Donut	12

Favorite Fatty Food Munchie	Fat Grams
Croissant	11
Slice of pizza	10
Large Dairy Queen ice cream dipped in chocolate	20
Dairy Queen banana split	15
Hot fudge sundae	26
Chocolate milkshake	10
Burger King regular onion rings	15
Burger King regular french fries	22
Hot dog	15
Corn dog	16
Dairy Queen super cheese dog	36
4 ounces refried beans with sausage	32
Jack in the Box super taco	17
Burger King double cheeseburger	32
Burger King Whopper	36
Burger King Whopper with cheese	45
Burger King double beef Whopper	52
Burger King double beef Whopper with cheese	62
Burger King Whopper Junior	20
Burger King Croissanwich with meat, egg, and cheese	24
Burger King ham and cheese sandwich	24
Arby's club sandwich	30
Arby's super roast beef sandwich	28
Arby's turkey sandwich	24
Arthur Treacher's fried fish	19.7
Arthur Treacher's fish sandwich	19.2
McDonald's Egg McMuffin	14
McDonald's Sausage McMuffin with egg	27.4

Favorite Fatty Food Munchie	Fat Grams
Taco Bell beef burrito	20
Wendy's baked potato with cheese	24
Wendy's baked potato plain	2 (for contrast)

(See pages 162–167 for replacement munchies.)

When you come to think of it, no wonder so many people gain weight when they go to college—even though they don't feel as if they're eating very much. In fact, they're *not* eating very much. They're just eating the wrong things.

HEALTH FOODS THAT AREN'T

One of the things that most dismays me is when I (Marthe) see a college student stuffing her face with foods such as sunflower seeds or granola bars in the false belief that she is eating a health food, when the fact is these foods have a very high fat content. From now on, the bottom line for you is, "When in doubt, leave it out," at least until you do some checking. In many cases, the food label itself will tell you the fat content. Other times, if it is not listed in this chapter as a food no-no and you are in doubt, you may have to look it up in a fat-gram counter.

WHERE WILL YOU GET YOUR DAILY TWENTY TO THIRTY GRAMS OF FAT?

Unlike protein and carbohydrates, you will not be given a list of specific foods to eat in order to get your twenty to thirty grams of fat per day. You will automatically consume your fat allowance in your protein requirement (and some of it in your carbohydrate allowance). In case you're wondering, however, it's okay to go below twenty grams of fat per day—even as low as fourteen grams, but as you will soon find out, that is very difficult to do.

Rule No. 2: Eat Two to Three Portions of Low-Fat Protein Per Day

Even the healthiest protein selections contain a fair amount of fat. So why not eliminate protein from your diet and just consume carbohydrates? You can't do it because the body relies heavily upon protein for its building and repair system. Protein is what muscle, blood, skin, hair, fingernails, immune cells, and internal organs are made of and are repaired by. Protein also affects the production of the hormones that control metabolism, growth, and sexual development, and it helps to regulate the acid-alkaline balance of the blood and tissues, as well as the body's water balance.

Unlike fat, protein cannot be stored, so we should eat protein in small portions spread throughout the day. The minimum amount of daily protein intake is forty-four grams per day, but since you will be building muscles, and muscles like a little more protein than that, you can consume up to one half a gram of protein per day for each pound you weigh. For example, if you weigh 130 pounds, you can consume sixty-five grams of protein per day.

WHERE WILL YOU GET YOUR PROTEIN ALLOWANCE?

You may consume your protein in chicken, turkey, fish, and nonmeat sources. But you must be careful to consume these without additional fat. For example, if you are having canned tuna, have tuna in water. If you are eating fish, be sure it is broiled or baked without butter. The same goes for chicken or turkey, choosing the white meat if possible and removing the skin.

POULTRY AND FISH SOURCES OF PROTEIN

Why remove skin from poultry and why not have it fried? Take a look at this:

4 Ounces Fast Food Fried Chicken	Fat Grams
Drumstick	16
Thigh	19
Breast	15

4 Ounces of Skinless, Broiled Chicken	Fat Grams
Drumstick	8
Thigh	9
Breast	5

4 Ounces of Skinless, Broiled Turkey	Fat Grams
Drumstick	4
Thigh	5
Breast	2

As you've probably observed, white meat poultry (breast) is the lowest in fat, and turkey is even lower in fat than chicken. There are about five grams of protein in every ounce of chicken, and about six grams in every ounce of turkey.

Most fish is relatively low in fat, but some fish is high and should be avoided until you reach your weight goal. They are:

6 Ounces Fish	Fat Grams
Swordfish	12
Salmon	11.1
Brook trout	6.3

You can choose from the following low-fat fish:

6 Ounces Fish	Fat Grams
Haddock	0.03
Red snapper	0.7
Cod	0.9
Abalone	0.9
Sea bass	1.5
Sole	2.4
Flounder	2.4
Squid	2.7
Tuna in water	3
Pike	3
Halibut	3.6
Scallops	4.2

There are about five grams of protein in every ounce of fish.

NONMEAT OR VEGETARIAN SOURCES OF PROTEIN

You may have cottage cheese, but make sure it's 1-percent fat, or no-fat. Look at the contrast:

1/2 Cup Cottage Cheese	Fat Grams
4 percent fat (creamed)	5.1
2 percent fat	2.2
1 percent fat	1.2
No-fat	0

There are about four grams of protein in every ounce of cottage cheese.

WHY CHEESE IS OUT OF THE QUESTION UNTIL YOU REACH YOUR GOAL

Take a look at this:

1 Ounce Regular Cheese	Fat Grams
Processed American	8.9
Cheddar	9.4
Colby	9.1
Edam	7.9
Feta	6
Gouda	7.8
Jarlsberg	6.9
Limburger	7.7
Monterey Jack	8.6

1 Ounce Regular Cheese	Fat Grams
Mozzarella	6.1
Muenster	8.5
Provolone	7.6
Roquefort	8.7
Swiss	7.8

If you eat three slices of cheese, you've already used up your fat limit for the day. For the same amount of fat, you could have eaten five full meals of nutritious foods and you would have felt satisfied.

LOW-FAT CHEESES

Forget about low-fat cheeses too. Even though they are lower in fat, there's still too much fat if you're trying to keep your fat grams low, because the problem is you're very unlikely to be satisfied with only one slice.

1 Ounce of Low-Fat Cheese	Fat Grams
Reduced-calorie American	2.2
Lite cheddar	3
Lite Swiss	3
Part-skim mozzarella	4.5

WHAT ABOUT PIZZA?

Pizza is a delicious, nutritious food, but because of its high cheese content you have to give it up until you reach your weight goal, unless you are in an emergency situation, and then you can blot it like a madwoman, and remove half the cheese.

Pizza	Fat Grams
2 slices Domino's cheese	10
1 slice Pizza Hut cheese pan pizza	18
2 slices Domino's pepperoni	18
1 Pizza Hut personal pan pepperoni	29

OTHER NONMEAT SOURCES OF PROTEIN

The following are excellent sources of low-fat protein. I (Marthe) live on yogurt.

Food	Fat Grams	Protein Grams
8 ounces low-fat yogurt	3.5	12
8 ounces no-fat yogurt	0	12
8 ounces 1 percent fat milk	2.6	8
8 ounces skim milk	0.4	8
1/2 cup beans	0.4	8
3 egg whites	0	10
1/2 cup tofu	4.5	8

PORTION SIZES OF PROTEIN

You will have two to three protein portions per day. One portion consists of:

6 ounces low-fat poultry or fish
1 cup low-fat skim milk
⅔ cup low-fat cottage cheese
1 cup low-fat yogurt
½ cup beans
½ cup tofu
3 egg whites (If you wish, you may have one yolk
scrambled with the whites. A yolk is 5.2 grams of fat.)

Since fish and poultry have about five grams of protein per ounce, and you are allowed six ounces per portion, you will get about thirty grams of protein in a portion, but other nonmeat sources supply half to one third that amount. So as a general rule, it's a good idea to have at least one of your protein portions in the fish-poultry category. If you do not, you can up your protein portions to three a day, or just eat less protein for that day. No big deal!

REPLACEMENT MUNCHIES:
FOODS THAT WILL NOT BLOW YOUR DIET

As you read rules 3 through 5, you will find a variety of foods that you can eat—some with limitation and others to your heart's content—foods that will not blow your diet. Get in the habit of keeping a generous supply of these foods available so that when you are cramming for an exam or just hanging around with friends, you don't put yourself in the position where you are forced to go off your diet because you are starving and there's nothing else to eat but the potato chips or donuts that your roommates have just brought in.

Rule No. 3: Eat Three to Five Portions of Limited Complex Carbohydrates a Day, and Two to Four Fruits a Day

Carbohydrates are broken down into two groups: simple carbohydrates (sugars), which themselves break down into two groups, processed and unprocessed (sugars are processed, and fruit is unprocessed), and complex carbohydrates such as vegetables, grains, and fiber. They are the best food bargain because they supply your body with a continual source of gradually released energy, and help you to never feel hungry. It is the complex carbohydrates listed here that you will reach for when you need energy to stay up all night cramming for an exam. As you read on, you will see which complex carbohydrates you can eat anytime you want to put something in your mouth, and which ones you can eat with limitation. You will also find out more about simple carbohydrates and why some are healthier than others.

Both simple and complex carbohydrates are the main source of energy for the body and the brain.

Limited complex carbohydrates are limited only because they are higher in calories than unlimited complex carbohydrates (to be discussed later).

Limited Complex Carbohydrates

½ bagel (or you can eat a whole bagel, using up two portions)
2 slices bread

1 ounce pretzels (a great munchie to replace potato chips)
1 English muffin
8 crackers
1 ounce dry cereal
4 ounces pasta (measured dry)
⅔ cup cooked rice
1 bowl hot or cold cereal
4 rice cakes
1 medium-large baked potato, sweet potato, or yam
1 cup corn or 1 large corn on the cob
½ cup beans or lentils of any kind
1 cup peas of any kind

ONCE IN A WHILE—JAM, JELLY, OR HARD SUGARY CANDY!

The least desirable simple carbohydrates are refined sugars found in candy and desserts (sucrose, fructose, lactose, dextrose, and others). Occasionally, to satisfy your sweet tooth, you can indulge in jam or jelly on whole wheat toast, or hard sugary candy. Limit this because such indulgences can trigger a hunger reaction and make you want to snack all day long. Also, too much sugar retards fat burning. So be careful with the straight sugars.

EAT TWO TO FOUR FRUITS PER DAY

Fruits are a much healthier source of simple carbohydrates. They are loaded with vitamins and fiber. They are also calorie dense (see below), and like all simple carbohydrates are an immediate source of energy.

Rule No. 4: To Prevent Constant Eating Due to Hunger, Choose Filling Foods That Are High in Caloric Density

Some foods are preferable to others because they are more filling, and will help you to resist the temptation to lose control, and in a fit of hunger put the wrong foods in your mouth. These foods are called calorie dense, because ounce for ounce they have fewer calories and more weight. Let me explain.

Since our stomachs can't hold more than two to three pounds of food, if we eat calorie dense foods, we will feel full by eating a small amount of calories. For example, you will feel full after eating only two baked potatoes and two cups of vegetables (two pounds of food) and you will only have consumed about 400 calories, but if you tried to fill your stomach with two pounds of bread, even if low-fat whole wheat bread, which is only forty-five calories a slice and is good for you, you will have consumed about 2,000 calories.

Calorie Dense Foods

Potatoes, sweet potatoes, yams
Pasta
Rice
Oatmeal (and other hot cereals)
All unlimited complex carbohydrates

We're not saying that you should completely deprive yourself of nutritious complex carbohydrates that are not calorie dense, all we are saying is if you choose them, you may still feel a little hungry. That's okay too, because you can always make it up with the calorie dense free, unlimited complex carbohydrates listed in the next section.

Rule No. 5: Never Go More Than Four to Five Hours without Eating or Your Metabolism Will Slow Down and You Will Hinder Your Weight Loss. Eat Unlimited Complex Carbohydrates Whenever You Are Hungry.

Many vegetables are so low in calories that you can virtually eat as much as you want without worrying about it. These will be your greatest source of replacement munchies. Use them between meals and even before bed. (For health purposes, you should eat at least two and a half cups of any combination of these vegetables per day, but it's even better if you eat more than that.)

Asparagus	Kale
Broccoli	Lettuce
Brussels sprouts	Mushrooms
Cabbage	Onions
Carrots	Peppers—red or green
Cauliflower	Radishes
Celery	Spinach
Collards	Sprouts
Cucumber	Summer squash
Eggplant	Tomatoes
Green or yellow beans	Zucchini

You can cut up these vegetables and carry them in little zip-lock plastic bags so that you don't get that starvation feeling between classes, or when you're hanging out with friends who are binging on cheese crackers and peanuts.

FIBER

You will get your fiber from foods that are in the simple and complex carbohydrate category, but mainly from the complex carbohydrates. There are two types of fiber: soluble fiber (found in oat bran, psyllium, fresh fruits and vegetables, and legumes), which can be digested by the body, and insoluble fiber (found in whole wheat, whole grains, celery, corn, corn bran, green beans, green leafy vegetables and potato skins, and brown rice), which cannot be digested by the body.

Soluble fiber helps to lower blood sugar and cholesterol levels. Insoluble fiber supplies the stool with needed volume and helps to prevent constipation and eventual colon and rectal cancer. But insoluble fiber has another benefit. Since it cannot be digested by the human body, it is eliminated without registering as calories. So when you eat a food with insoluble fiber, you can automatically take off about 15 percent of the calorie content. In addition, when such a food exits the body, some of the fat in your digestive system clings to the rough surface of the fiber, and as the fiber exits the body, it pulls the fat along with it. In this sense, fiber serves, to some extent, as a fat vacuum.

HOW MUCH FIBER SHOULD YOU CONSUME EACH DAY?

The recommended daily allowance for fiber is about thirty grams per day. Here are the fiber counts for some foods.

Food	Fiber Grams
Grains	
1 ounce Kellogg's All-Bran with extra fiber	14
Fiber One (General Mills)	13
1 ounce bran flakes–type cereal	9
1 slice whole wheat bread	2
1 slice cracked wheat bread	2
1 slice rye bread	1
Fruits	
1 orange	5
1 pear	5
1 banana	4
1 cup strawberries	5
1 apple	3.5
Fresh Vegetables (*For one cup of each.*)	
Spinach	11
Peas	8
Corn	8
Broccoli	8
Carrots	5
Eggplant	5
Cabbage	4
Green beans	5
Tomato	4
Baked potato	6

Food	Fiber Grams

Beans and Legumes (*These are rich sources of fiber. For one cup.*)

Food	Fiber Grams
Baked beans	21
Split peas	21
Lentils	18

A lack of fiber in the diet causes constipation and eventual development of hemorrhoids—which can be both painful and embarrassing, so even if you're not impressed by the fact that fiber helps to prevent colon cancer and a host of other diseases, it's a good idea to make sure you include a healthy dose of fiber in your diet.

Salt Can't Make You Fat, but It Can Make You Retain Water and Cause You to Carry Temporary Weight—You May Feel Fat!

Sodium is a necessary mineral. It is used by the body to help regulate body fluids and maintain the acid-alkali balance of the blood. It is also responsible for muscle contraction.

You don't have to watch your sodium (salt) intake for this eating plan, but since sodium holds about fifty times its own weight in water, if you eat high-sodium foods (such as Chinese food that is loaded with MSG, a type of sodium), you will probably carry around from three to seven pounds of water.

Even though this water is a temporary weight gain, and can be eliminated by dropping your sodium intake, it can discourage you if you're dieting, because it may make you feel bloated and fat. Sometimes when people feel this way, they are tempted to say, "I might as well pig out, I'm as fat as a hog no matter what I do," and they not only start eating everything in sight—they stop working out. What a shame, because if they realized that the fat feeling was only temporary water retention, they could have ignored it and kept up with the plan.

Other people don't care if they carry around a few pounds of water, as long as it's not bathing suit season. They love salty foods, and if they have no problem with high blood pressure, they indulge in them until it is time to show off their bodies. They know that when they cut their sodium intake, the excess water will go—and they do just that when they want to show off their bodies on the beach or elsewhere.

You can make your own decision as to how much water weight you are willing to carry, but for your information, if you keep your sodium intake to between 1,500 and 2,500 milligrams daily, you probably won't retain water.

WHERE'S THE SALT?

High-sodium foods include all canned, smoked, and pickled foods, as well as Chinese food containing MSG, condiments such as ketchup, mustard, A-1, and other steak sauces, pizza, frankfurters, and fast foods in general, and diet frozen dinners. Most of the above have 1,000 milligrams of sodium or more per serving. By contrast, other foods contain:

Food (3 1/2 ounces)	Milligrams of Sodium
Chicken	60
Lettuce	4
Peas	1 (canned: 250)
Potatoes	3
Eggplant	2

Drinking Water Helps to Flush Out Your System

Water is the primary carrier of nutrients throughout the body, and is involved in nearly every body function, including absorption, digestion, and excretion (if you are dehydrated, you may become constipated because it is water that keeps food moving through the intestinal tract until it is eliminated). Water also helps circulation and body lubrication, and helps to regulate your body temperature.

More than half our body weight is water. A person could live for forty days without food—but could not live more than five days without water.

We use up about three quarts of water a day through perspiration, excretion, and even breathing. Most people replace this water through foods (fruit is 85 percent water, for example) and beverages such as soda, coffee, milk, soup, and juice, but do not go out of their way to drink plain old water.

Is it good enough to replace the three quarts of lost water through the above sources? Yes and no. While it is true that your body will not dehydrate as long as you replace it with a substantial amount of liquid, it will not be as happy with the above liquids as it would be if in addition you provided it with about six glasses of plain old water—whether it be tap or bottled. Think of it this way. Drinking plain water is the only way you can give your internal organs a clean shower. Bathing them in coffee, soup, and soda just isn't the same thing!

In order to insure that you do not retain water, it's a good idea to drink between six and eight eight-ounce glasses of water a day because water flushes out the excess sodium from your system.

WATER HELPS TO IMPROVE YOUR COMPLEXION AND CURB YOUR APPETITE

You can space your water out systematically by drinking a glass when you wake up, one before each meal, and one before bedtime. You will notice that once you start drinking lots of water your complexion will improve. In a matter of days, your skin will have a healthier color and will seem to glow.

Water also helps to curb your appetite. Did you know that many times when you think you are hungry, you are really only thirsty, but because your body knows that you are not going to give it water, it leads you to water-filled, and sometimes fat-filled, foods?

What About Beer and Hard Liquor?

Although beer (even regular beer, not the light) and hard liquor have virtually no fat (unless you choose mixed drinks made with milk or cream), it is easy enough to gain weight on them—if you drink to excess.

What is excess? If you're trying to lose weight and get in shape, anything more than three or four beers or glasses of wine, or two or three shots of hard liquor per week is in excess. Why? Setting aside health concerns for the moment, drink calories add up very quickly—and even though carbohydrate calories (found in beers, wines, and liquors) are not nearly as bad as fat calories (for reasons discussed above), if you consume enough of them, they add up to an amount your body will not be able to burn, and your body will have to store them as fat.

For example, if you drink six beers in one night—a very bad idea because it will dull your brain as well as make you fat—you will have consumed 600 calories if the beer is light, and 900 calories if it's regular. Do this five nights a week, and you've consumed 3,000 or 4,500 calories. For every 3,500 excess calories you consume, you store one pound of fat.

So you see, you could be gaining a pound a week in college just on the beer you've been drinking, if you've been drinking to excess!

If you are going to do any drinking, however, it's important that you follow the basic guideline of sticking to light beer or hard liquor mixed only with no-calorie sodas or fruit juice. Why double the damage?

Participating without Feeling Deprived

Even though it will take a little thinking ahead, if you take care of yourself by making the necessary preparations (bringing your own plastic bags of food to your friend's room on all-nighter cramming sessions) and by thinking ahead (planning in advance what you will drink if you go to a bar), if you do it, you will be able to participate fully in the social scene at college without feeling deprived. The fact is there's no need to hide in your room and be a hermit just because you are losing weight. You can be out there in the middle of the action if you have a plan. And soon you'll get a break and be able to eat whatever you want one day a week.

When You Reach Your Goal: A Free Weekly Eating Day

Once you reach your goal, you can eat anything you want, all day long, once a week. Yes. You read correctly. As long as you observe the food guidelines in this chapter on the other six days of the week, you will be fine. In fact, you really should take advantage of the free eating day—don't refuse to do it out of fear.

Food should not become an obsessive thought to you. It should be a natural part of life. If you have to give up your favorite "naughty" foods forever, you would wait until a day you were very angry at yourself or the world, and then you would binge until you got fat, just to get even. If you know that nothing is forbidden to you, and that once you reach your goal you can look forward to a vacation from careful eating one day a week, you will no longer use food as a weapon against yourself.

PICKING AND CHOOSING FROM YOUR SCHOOL'S CAFETERIA MENU

Campus menus are notorious for offering a variety of high-fat foods, not just for dinner, but for breakfast and lunch as well. If you don't know what you're doing, it will be easy to consume three to five times your recommended fat allowance. But now that you know exactly what you're doing, that won't happen.

Let's look at one meal at a time.

Breakfast

A typical college menu offers:

Scrambled eggs
Sunny-side up eggs
Bacon
Hash brown potatoes
Waffles or pancakes and syrup
Croissant
Blueberry muffins, corn muffins, bran muffins
English muffins, bagels, toast
Hot and cold cereals
Cream cheese, jelly, butter
Cocoa, chocolate milk, full-fat milk
Coffee, tea, low-fat milk, skim milk
Apple juice, orange juice, grapefruit juice
Apples, oranges, peaches, pears

After having read this chapter, you might have guessed that the eggs are out—not so much because each egg yolk contains about six grams of fat, but because the eggs offered are prepared in fat—butter, margarine, or oil (margarine and oil have less cholesterol, but they have just as much fat as butter and will make you just as fat if you consume them).

Let's use butter as the example. One tablespoon of butter has 12.3 grams of fat, and chances are, by the time your scrambled eggs soak up the fat, you have 24.6 grams of fat. You've already used up your ideal fat allowance for the day. Sunny-side up eggs will probably soak up about one tablespoon of fat (12.3 grams). What a waste. And this is not even counting the two yolks—another 12 grams of fat! And who eats scrambled or sunny-side up eggs by themselves? Most people butter a slice or two of toast—another 12.3 grams of fat for sure.

If your school offers hard-boiled or poached eggs with no butter, you can have up to four per week. The American Heart Association recommends this limit because of the 213 milligrams of cholesterol (a potentially artery-clogging substance) in each yolk. Notice that it is the yolk that is limited, since whites have no fat at all, but are made of protein and have virtually no calories. Egg whites can be consumed without limit, and are an excellent source of protein.

What about bacon or hash browns? You already know that bacon is on the forbidden list. It has up to eighteen grams of fat per slice, so forget it. Hash browns would be great if they were made without butter or fat (plain potatoes, baked or boiled, have zero fat), but they are, so you can count on about twenty-four grams of fat there.

A medium serving of waffles or pancakes has up to fifteen grams of fat in them. Then if you put butter on them . . . (The syrup is not the problem. It has no fat—but it is made of pure sugar. Save your sugar for an occasional tablespoon of jam or jelly on your toast.)

The seemingly innocent croissant, as light and airy as it is, has eleven grams of fat—and once you develop a fat detector in your taste buds, you will immediately notice it as you bite into one. "Yuck, greasy," you will think.

SO, WHAT CAN YOU EAT FOR BREAKFAST?

Muffins (blueberry, bran, or corn) have about 4.5 grams of fat each. Not so bad for once in a while. English muffins, bagels, and regular whole wheat or white bread have about a gram of fat—excellent choice. You can spread a tablespoon of jam or jelly on these items (no fat in jam or jelly and only eighteen calories per teaspoon or fifty-four calories per tablespoon), or better yet, eat them plain. You already know why you must skip the butter or cream cheese.

Hot cereals, such as oatmeal, Cream of Wheat, Wheatena, and so on, have virtually no fat, but you must assume that they were prepared with full-fat milk. There won't be more than one fourth cup of milk in them, so you can count on only two grams of fat there. No problem. You can afford that. But if you add extra milk, make sure it's low-fat or skim—if your college has it. Otherwise, don't add milk.

Cold cereals vary—but not so much in their fat content, which is usually under a gram per bowl, except for Cap'n Crunch, which has 3.4 grams per cup, and Cracklin' Oat Bran, which has 3.0 grams—look at the box.

Cereals also vary a great deal in their fiber content. A general rule for choosing cereals is the less sugar and the more fiber the better. (See pages 167–169 for fiber guidelines.)

Most schools today are getting at least partially wise to the need to lower the fat in their cafeteria menus and offer low-fat or skim milk. Use this in your cereal, as well as in your coffee or tea, or even drink it plain.

Cocoa and chocolate milk are out because they can

contain between eight and fifteen grams of fat per glass—unless they are no- or low-fat, and most colleges don't offer such items yet.

Although it's better to eat a piece of fruit than to drink a glass of juice, because the fruit contains more fiber and is more filling, you may have a small glass of juice once in a while if you wish. (Juice contains no fat, and a six-ounce glass can be counted as one fruit.)

Lunch

A typical college menu offers:

Hamburgers, cheeseburgers, fries
Sandwiches: ham and cheese, roast beef, corned beef,
tuna salad, chicken salad
Macaroni and cheese
Mashed potatoes, Tater Tots, fried potatoes
Steak-ums, fish sticks
Turkey and gravy
Barbecue chicken
Vegetables with butter
Soup
Salad bar
Corn on the cob, baked potato
Brown, wild, yellow, or white rice
Yogurt
Fruit
Soda, orange drink, juice, diet soda

Not easy pickings if you're trying to keep your fat intake low. You already know that hamburgers, cheeseburgers, ham and cheese, roast beef, and corned beef are out of the question (too much fat, and so are on the Fat Bandit list, see page 153).

Tuna and chicken salad would be fine—if there were no mayonnaise added (eleven grams of fat per tablespoon).

Macaroni and cheese is out because of the cheese, and mashed potatoes, Tater Tots, and fried potatoes are out because they are made with butter or some form of fat.

Steak-ums are out because beef is too high in fat, and fish sticks are out because they are breaded and fried in fat.

WHAT CAN YOU EAT FOR LUNCH?

Turkey is okay if you scrape off the gravy. Barbecue chicken is fine if you remove the skin and scrape off the barbecue sauce, and try to eat more of the white meat than the dark.

Unfortunately, most colleges still saturate the vegetables in butter, but if you don't mind people looking at you, you can eat them if you place them onto a few napkins and blot off most of the butter.

Soups are okay if they are chicken, turkey, vegetable, minestrone, tomato, pea, mushroom, onion, or clam chowder—*if* they are not creamed (made with milk or cream). If not creamed, these soups have one to three grams of fat per cup—a real fat bargain—and a hot bowl of soup can be very satisfying.

The salad bar can either save your diet life or kill it, depending upon whether or not you know what you're doing. You can fill up on raw vegetables such as tomatoes, lettuce, broccoli, cauliflower, radishes, sprouts, and so on. But don't add any dressing at all. Trust me. It's all fat: about eight grams of fat a tablespoon is average, and you will probably use at least four tablespoons, for a whopping thirty-two grams of fat. If you want to, you can buy a bottle of plain wine vinegar and carry it in your bag. You can pour it over the salad and have a fine treat.

The bean salads in the salad bar would be great, but they are always made with oil, so forget it. The cottage cheese would be great, but you can count on it being full-fat (five grams of fat for one half cup). You can have it, but don't forget to count it into your fat allowance for the day.

The bottom line on the salad bar is: use it intelligently!

Corn on the cob and baked potatoes are excellent food choices, as long as you don't put any butter on them. You can settle for a little table salt on the corn, and perhaps some low-fat yogurt (if your college offers it) on the baked potato as a substitute for sour cream or butter.

Rice of any kind is great—*if* it is not prepared with butter or oil—and in most college cafeterias it usually is. It is more difficult to get the butter off rice than vegetables, since rice absorbs butter quickly, so unless your cafeteria dietitian says the rice is prepared without butter or oil, stay away from it.

Yogurt is a lifesaver—if it is low- or no-fat. Most low-fat yogurts, flavored or otherwise, have no more than three grams of fat per cup. Frozen low-fat yogurt has about four grams of fat per serving (one half cup). It's okay to have one serving, but since frozen low-fat yogurt is so delicious, it would be tempting to have three servings, and then you would have consumed twelve grams of fat. So use self-discipline in this area. No-fat yogurt of any kind has virtually no fat, but keep dreaming if you think your college cafeteria is going to offer it. (If they do, please write to me at the P.O. Box on page 190. I would love to know.)

But what if your cafeteria is still living in the dark ages, and offers only full-fat yogurt? There are about 7.4 grams of fat per cup. I say it's not worth it, but in an emergency, once in a while, okay.

Fruit is probably the safest no-fat item on the college campus.

Choose seltzer over club soda (less sodium), and diet

soda over regular soda (fewer calories), and choose juice over fruit drinks (juice has vitamins and nutrients, while fruit drinks have sugar). You may also drink plain water— dare I say, if they have it!

If the lunch menu is really limited, you can always resort to cold cereal, or you could bring a whole wheat pita shell and some vinegar, and stuff it with a variety of legitimate pickings from the salad bar, or bring a can of tuna in water and a couple of slices of whole wheat bread. The key is: if you think ahead, you can survive.

Dinner

A typical college menu offers:

Pork chops, steak, veal cutlets, meatballs, sausages, ham
Fried chicken, fried fish
Broiled turkey, broiled chicken, broiled fish
Mashed potatoes, dumplings
Egg noodles with butter, fried rice
Vegetables, stir-fry Chinese vegetables
Baked ziti, lasagna, pizza
Pasta with meat sauce, pasta with tomato sauce
Salad bar (see above)
Beverages (see above)

It looks bad, but all is not lost. After we immediately eliminate the obvious fat bandits: pork chops, steak, veal cutlets, meatballs, sausages, and ham, we can work with the fried chicken and fish, as I'll discuss below.

Egg noodles with butter and fried rice are out of the question. Both food items absorb fats quickly, and you would have to take each individual noodle or rice grain and blot out the fat. (Egg noodles are always a waste of fat grams, since they are made with fatty egg yolks. You could get the same delicious taste, or better, with plain noodles not made from egg!)

Baked ziti and lasagna are also out of the question because they contain too much cheese. Pizza has too much cheese for your purposes, but in an emergency if you remove half the cheese and then blot the pizza to remove most of the excess oil, you could have it because you would be cutting the fat by at least half.

WHAT CAN YOU EAT FOR DINNER?

You can remove any skin from the fried chicken, and then blot it thoroughly with a napkin. Gently squeeze the chicken completely between three napkins until all excess grease is absorbed by the napkins. Fried fish is a little more difficult, because it absorbs grease more quickly than does chicken, but you can get at least 75 percent of it off by blotting and gently squeezing.

The broiled turkey, chicken, and fish are perfect—assuming the cooks didn't blow the whole thing by saturating the foods with butter. If they did, again, blot away!

Dumplings are a possibility, because fat is usually not a big ingredient in them, but is rather put on top of them (usually in the gravy). If you can get the dumplings plain, okay. Vegetables and stir-fry Chinese vegetables can be blotted to remove butter and grease. Use the old napkin trick.

By now, you might be thinking, "Are you kidding. I wouldn't blot my food in front of everyone. People will look at me and think I'm a real ..." But think of this: Are those people going to help you when you keep putting on weight day after day? Are they going to comfort you when you're getting dressed to go out and you can't zip up your jeans? Are they going to keep buying you "fat clothes" to hide your figure, and are they going to magically take the weight off you when it becomes too much to bear? Of course not! So let them look away while you blot away. And in a few months, they'll be looking toward you for advice on how to get in shape, because you'll look gorgeous, and what's more, you'll feel so much better about yourself.

If tomato sauce is not available, you can have a small portion (one serving) of pasta with meat sauce, because meat sauces only contain a small amount of fat. Pasta with tomato sauce is of course much better, since it has almost no fat at all.

If a salad bar is available, use it as discussed in the lunch menu. Beverages should be used as discussed in the above paragraphs.

SURVIVAL TECHNIQUES FOR COLLEGE CAFETERIA EATING

Survival techniques 1 and 2 have already been discussed. They are:

Survival Technique No. 1: Pick and choose wisely from the cafeteria menu

Survival Technique No. 2: Blot foods cooked in butter or grease in a few napkins

Now it's time to discuss survival technique No. 3, which was for me (Marthe) a lifesaver, especially when I attended Fairfield University where the menu was nearly impossible.

Survival Technique No. 3: Keep a supply of low-fat foods in your room

Ideally, you should have your own small refrigerator, but if you don't, there is still a lot you can do. First we'll discuss foods you can use if no refrigerator is available (these of course also apply to those who have a refrigerator). Then we'll discuss what to get when a refrigerator is available.

NO REFRIGERATOR

The following food items will save your life:

Cold cereals and powdered low-fat milk
Envelopes of instant oatmeal or other cereal (you can
cook them up with hot tap water)
Cans of tuna in water
Boxes of instant rice that can be made with hot (tap) or
boiled water
Whole wheat bread, bagels, English muffins, pretzels
Jam or jelly if you can handle it—or no-sugar jam or
jelly if you can't
Raw vegetables and fruit that keeps (carrots and celery,
apples or grapefruit, for example)
Bottled water, diet soda, herbal teas

REFRIGERATOR

All vegetables and fruits
Low- or no-fat yogurt and cottage cheese
Eggs (for the whites)
White meat chicken and turkey
Potatoes (you can boil them if you have a pot, or
microwave them if you have one—but many dorms do
not allow these items)

If possible, keep a microwave, a toaster, and an electric
pot in your room. These items can be lifesavers.

Making Up Your Daily Menu—
How Strict Are the Rules?

Most of the previously discussed rules are simply guidelines. You don't have to eat two to three portions of low-fat protein per day. Eating three to five limited complex carbohydrates is not a must. You don't have to eat two to four fruits per day. You don't have to eat at least two and one half cups of free, unlimited complex carbohydrates a day. But try to keep within the guidelines, because if you generally do, not only will you lose maximum fat, but you will have high energy and be in the best of health.

A few of the rules, however, are musts. Eating often *is* a must, to keep your metabolism going. Keeping your fat between twenty and thirty grams a day is also a must. Doing the College Dorm Workout is also a must.

Use This Code Card to Remind You!

Make up a code card and keep it handy so you will remember the general rules. Here is a sample code card:

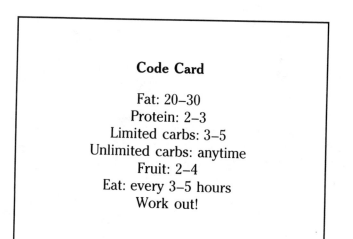

Code Card

Fat: 20–30
Protein: 2–3
Limited carbs: 3–5
Unlimited carbs: anytime
Fruit: 2–4
Eat: every 3–5 hours
Work out!

Read through this chapter a couple of times, highlighting the important facts, and every so often skim through the chapter and review the highlighted areas. Soon the information and tips will be permanently in your mind.

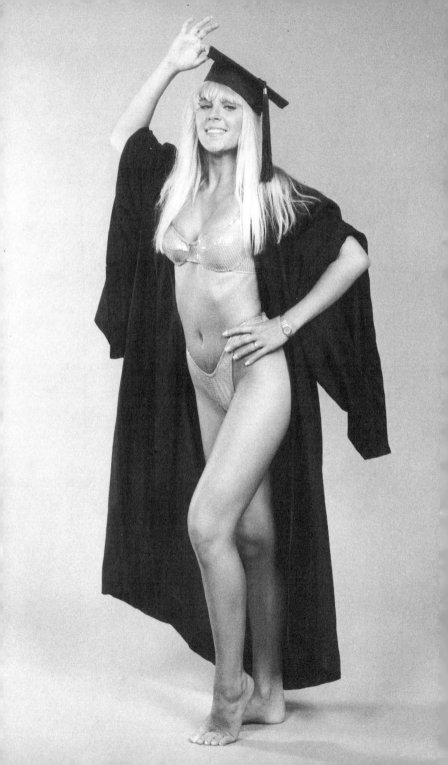

THE FINAL WORD

You don't have to get fat just because you're in college and the menu is impossible. Even if you keep no food in your room—refrigerator or otherwise, by following the cafeteria eating suggestions, you can survive. True, it does take some effort, and in fact, at first it may seem like a big hassle. But after you get used to it, you won't think twice about it, and what's more important, you'll begin to see an amazing difference in your body.

After I gained almost fifteen pounds in my first semester, I started using the methods described in this book. Then, slowly but surely, pound by pound (sometimes I lost nothing in one week, other times I lost two pounds, still other times I lost a fraction of a pound, and sometimes the scale even went up a pound—I guess it was water weight), the excess weight came off and I was able to stop obsessing about my body. But what was much more important than just losing the excess weight, with the College Dorm Workout I was able to make my body tight and toned—hard and defined instead of soft and mushy.

There's no substitute for muscles in all the right places—and they're really not that difficult to acquire, if you're consistent, and more important, if you do it right. This book shows you how to do it right. In fact, it's literally impossible *not* to get a tight, toned, muscular body if you follow this workout for ten weeks. Take it from me and thousands of other college students who have tried it. It works. Be sure to take a before photograph of yourself, and then one in ten weeks. Send me the results!

Also, if you have a question or comment, feel free to write to me. Enclose a stamped, self-addressed envelope if you wish a reply. Address your letter to:

Marthe S. Vedral
P.O. Box A 433
Wantagh, NY 11793-0433

TO ORDER
CAST-IRON DUMBBELLS

Set of five-pound dumbbells: $17.98, plus $8.52 shipping and handling.
   Total: $26.50

Set of three-pound dumbbells: $12.98, plus $6.52 shipping and handling.
   Total: $19.50

Send a check or money order to:

Marthe S. Vedral
P.O. Box A 433
Wantagh, NY 11793-0433

BIBLIOGRAPHY

Katahan, Martin, Ph.D., and Jamioe Pope-Curdle, M.S., R.D. *The T-Factor Fat Gram Counter.* New York: W.W. Norton & Company, 1989.

Kneuer, Cameo, and Joyce L. Vedral, Ph.D. *Cameo Fitness.* New York: Warner Books, 1990.

McLish, Rachel, and Joyce L. Vedral, Ph.D. *Perfect Parts.* New York: Warner Books, 1987.

Vedral, Joyce, Ph.D. *Bottoms Up.* New York: Warner Books, 1993.

———. *The Fat-Burning Workout.* New York: Warner Books, 1991. (For video call 1-800-433-6769.)

———. *Gut Busters.* New York: Warner Books, 1992.

———. *Now or Never.* New York: Warner Books, 1986.

———. *The Twelve-Minute Total-Body Workout.* New York: Warner Books, 1989.

INDEX